Award-winning writer, television broadcaster and author of numerous bestsellers, **Leslie Kenton** is described by the press as 'the guru of health and fitness' and 'the most original voice in health'. A shining example of energy and commitment, she is highly respected for her thorough reporting. Leslie was born in California, and is the daughter of jazz musician Stan Kenton. After leaving Stanford University she journeyed to Europe in her early twenties, settling first in Paris then in Britain where she has since remained. She has raised four children on her own by working as a television broadcaster, novelist, writer and teacher on health and for fourteen years she was an editor at *Harpers & Queen*.

Leslie's writing on mainstream health is internationally known and has appeared in *Vogue*, the *Sunday Times*, *Cosmopolitan* and the *Daily Mail*. She is the author of many other health books including: *The New Raw Energy* and *Raw Energy Recipes* – co-authored with her daughter Susannah – *The New Ultrahealth*, *The New Joy of Beauty*, *The New Ageless Ageing*, *Cellulite Revolution*, *10 Day Clean-Up Plan*, *Endless Energy*, *Nature's Child*, *Lean Revolution* and the *10 Day De-Stress Plan*. She turned to fiction with *Ludwig* – her first novel. Former consultant to a medical corporation in the USA and to the Open University's Centre of Continuing Education, Leslie's writing has won several awards including the PPA 'Technical Writer of the Year'. Her work was honoured by her being asked to deliver the McCarrison Lecture at the Royal Society of Medicine. In recent years she has become increasingly concerned not only with the process of enhancing individual health but also with re-establishing bonds with the earth as a part of helping to heal the planet.

THE NEW
BIOGENIC DIET

The ultimate guide to weight-loss through food combining

LESLIE KENTON

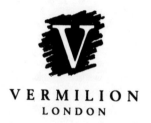

VERMILION
LONDON

1 3 5 7 9 10 8 6 4 2

First published in the United Kingdom in 1995 by
Vermilion
an imprint of Ebury Press
Random House
20 Vauxhall Bridge Road
London SW1V 2SA

Random House Australia (Pty) Limited
20 Alfred Street, Milsons Point, Sydney,
New South Wales 2061, Australia

Random House New Zealand Limited
18 Poland Road, Glenfield,
Auckland 10, New Zealand

Random House South Africa (Pty) Limited
PO Box 337, Bergvlei, South Africa

Random House Canada
1265 Aerowood Drive, Mississauga,
Ontario L4W 1B9, Canada

Random House UK Limited Reg. No. 954009

A CIP catalogue record for this book is available from the
British Library

ISBN: 0 09 178444 1

Photoset by Deltatype Ltd, Ellesmere Port
Printed and bound in Great Britain by Cox & Wyman
Ltd, Reading, Berkshire

Papers used by Ebury Press are natural recyclable
products made from wood grown in sustainable forests.

For Dr Cindy Buttoo
with admiration and affection

Acknowledgements

Many physicians and scientists have contributed to make this book possible. So have a number of conscientious and successful slimmers determined once and for all to shed their unwanted fat. It would be impossible to thank them all properly. There are a few to whom I am particularly indebted: Ralph Bircher, Dagmar Liechte von Brasch, Phillip Kilsby, Doris Grant, Bob Erdmann, Gordon and Barbara Latto, Keki Sidwah, I. I. Brekhman, Robert O. Becker, John Douglass, Henning Karstrom, Fritz Popp, and Herbert Pohl. I am especially grateful to Graham Jones who spent several sleepless nights in front of the word processor recording my corrections and who gave such positive support when I most needed it.

Leslie Kenton
Pembrokeshire 1995

Contents

Foreword to the First Edition

Leslie Kenton was elected 'Technical Writer of the Year' because of her impeccable accuracy in reporting scientific information combined with a clarity of expression that gives her writing a sense of thrill and excitement at the discoveries in the field of science and their intelligent application for the wellbeing of all of us. In this volume she has successfully tackled the subject of weight-loss, in terms of both its physiology and its psychology, and has brought the ancient concept of biogenic living into 1986 for the special benefit of those who need to shed excess fat.

We are delighted to have been asked to write this foreword because we have long been familiar with Székely's rediscovery of biogenic or life-promoting principles, and feel than no one could better present these ideas to the lay reader than Leslie Kenton. Moreover, she is not writing purely as a disinterested reporter: she practises what she preaches in the field of nutrition, exercise, relaxation, meditation and all that goes with them.

Biogenics is much more than just a way of losing weight. It has wide implications for the physical, mental and spiritual health of us all. It is pleasing to see that Leslie has not ignored these.

We have known Leslie and her delightful children since 1970, long before she became so well known. Her outstanding capacity for hard work is matched by her capacity for caring and loving. She has a strong sense of responsibility for life which is reflected in everything she writes. We wish the book 'God Speed'.

Drs Gordon and Barbara Latto

Author's Note

This is a book about biogenics – a way of eating and living which can rid your body of excess fat deposits permanently without your needing to count calories. It is not about illness and how to cure it. The material in this book is intended for informational purposes only. None of the suggestions or information is meant in any way to be prescriptive. Any attempt to treat a medical condition should always come under the direction of a competent physician or health practitioner who is familiar with nutritional therapy and neither the publisher nor I can accept responsibility for injuries or illness arising out of a failure by a reader to take medical advice. I am only a reporter, although one who has for many years sought a method of permanent fat-loss which would heighten energy levels, help protect from premature ageing and from illness and make me look good and feel great. In biogenics I found it. I write in the simple hope that some of what I have learned may be of use to others.

The word 'biogenic' was first coined by Edmond Bordeaux Székely. He used the word to describe the 'life-generating' properties of living embryonic foods such as sprouted seeds and grains and baby greens. Székely also coined the word 'biocidic' to mean foods which are 'life-destroying' – namely flesh foods and highly processed foods containing chemicals etc. Székely founded the International Biogenic Society (Apartado 372, Cartago, Costa Rica) which despite his death continues with unabated enthusiasm to teach his excellent methods for living and healing in harmony with Nature's laws and the earth's living energies. I have borrowed his excellent words but here you will find them used in a somewhat different way (see pages 31-33). For instance, Székely would never suggest that anyone eat flesh foods of any kind, while they do form a small part of the way of eating outlined in this book. This I have done because I believe that for most people living in the late twentieth-century urban environment it is too great a change to make all at once to switch from our usual Western diet to one as strict as Székely suggests. I very much hope however that for at least some of my readers *The New Biogenic Diet* will serve as an interim step that will eventually take them closer and closer to Székely's ideals (see page 246 for a full list of his books and publications).

PART ONE

THE PRINCIPLES

1
Lean and Alive

AN OVER-FAT BODY is an unhealthy body. It is more inclined than a lean one to premature ageing and more likely to develop a degenerative disease such as coronary heart disease, diabetes, arthritis or cancer. Even more important, such a body never experiences its full potential for vitality, energy and joy at simply being alive because it is unable to live at a high level of wellbeing.

Real health cannot be measured by the absence of disease alone. It goes far beyond. And it is not so much a *state* as a living *process* – a process through which you can make greater and greater use of your innate potential for creativity, aliveness and joy.

Have you ever seen a young horse racing from one end of his field to another for the sheer pleasure of the feeling of movement in his body? Watching him move with dilated nostrils and mane blowing free can give you a real sense of what a high level of wellbeing – health in its broadest sense – is all about: ease, freedom and, above all, *aliveness.*

Few overweight people experience such aliveness no matter how so-called 'healthy' they are. I know. I myself have been one of those 'healthy' overweights and it isn't fun. Like many other people who have carried from 10 to 50 (or even more) pounds of excess fat about on their frame, I have many times wanted to move as the horse does – to run with energy and joy just because it feels good to be alive and to have a sense of strength and freedom of movement in my body. And many times I have had to settle for second-best – lumbering more like a self-conscious rhinoceros and faintly hoping that nobody would notice the great effort it all took or remark on the gracelessness of my movements.

Unfortunately, no matter how much you console yourself with the idea that you are generally healthy, that you eat well, that you have genetically inherited a tendency to be fat or that the latest statistics reassuringly indicate you can be considerably over the insurance statistic weight charts and still be 'safe', most of us who are or have ever been over-fat have a sense that to some extent we are missing out. We are not as alive as we could be, nor as beautiful, nor as joyous – and we know it.

Make Way for Biogenics

Biogenic food combining can change that for you. It has for me and thousands of other people who have used it either because they are resistant to weight-loss or generally less healthy than they could be. The word 'biogenic' means life-generating. It describes a unique approach to health, nutrition and permanent weight-loss based on natural fresh foods which have been carefully combined. We will be exploring the biogenic system in depth in the chapters which follow.

'Biogenics' is an apt name for this superbly effective way of eating and living which can enhance cellular vitality, help restore healthy metabolism and normal weight, and encourage your body to rebalance its biophysical and biochemical functioning so you are able to live at a high level of energy and 'aliveness'.

Just in case you are worried that what you will be reading is some newfangled idea, rest assured. There is little new about biogenics. Nor can I take much credit for what follows. I am only a reporter – someone who discovered biogenics because I myself went searching for a solution to my own fat-shedding challenge. I learned about it as a result of ploughing through literally hundreds of books and scientific papers and talking to scores of physicians, biochemists and natural health practitioners who have used it in one form or another for trimming down their patients and for encouraging the bodies of unwell people to heal themselves. That, after all, is what permanent fat-loss is all about – restoring normal functioning and form to a body which has become unbalanced, sluggish, and distorted in size, texture and shape.

Living Sculpture

Michelangelo claimed that he never imposed any shape or form onto the piece of marble he was carving. He insisted that instead he simply used his sculptor's tools to *reveal the natural form hidden within* the marble. In many ways your overweight body is rather like his marble. Within it is hidden its vital, naturally healthy and lean form. Biogenics is nothing more than an efficient tool for helping you uncover it – a biological method of 'living sculpture'.

The idea that steady and permanent fat-loss can take place the biogenic way – as a result of eating natural delicious foods at specific times of the day, avoiding certain food combinations, and getting regular but non-strenuous exercise – may come as a shock to some people, both nutritionists and laymen alike, who have been brought up to believe that counting calories and going hungry is the *only* way to shed excess weight. I have even seen it make a few 'dedicated calorie-counters' very angry indeed. For old assumptions about weight-loss die hard. And as you might imagine biogenics is decidedly unpopular with the multi-million-pound slimming industry, which survives on people's failures – failures which keep diet products selling almost as fast as they can be manufactured. But it can be a godsend to people who, like me, have struggled for a long time with the battle of the bulge and who genuinely want to get rid of fat which does not rightly belong to them, and to 'run free' as the horse does.

As Old as Civilization

A system of living based on natural fresh foods – vegetables and fruits, wholegrains, seeds and nuts and dairy products with fish, poultry and game if you wish – biogenics has been used with minor variations, depending upon culture and custom, for healing and for enhancing mental and physical awareness throughout the civilized world for quite literally thousands of years. Hippocrates, the father of modern medicine, who said 'let your foods be your medicine', knew about it, as did the famous European physician Paracelsus in the Middle Ages. The Essenes who lived in the Holy Land at the time of Jesus based all their teachings about mental and physical health on a biogenic way of life. It also formed the foundation of treatment for doctors who were part of what in the nineteenth century was known as the 'natural hygiene movement' in the United States and Britain. In Paris during the 1920s French author and

Nobel laureate Romain Rolland together with Edmond Székely formed what they called the International Biogenic Society for Living – a group of people throughout the world intent on exploring the use of biogenic principles for enhancing health. Biogenic principles also form the basis of health and rejuvenation treatment at many of Europe's and America's finest spas.

Perfect Mix

The biogenic diet also asks that you pay attention to the particular way in which foods are *combined* to encourage natural fat-loss even in the most resistant bodies. This category includes women with cellulite, people whose metabolism has been drastically slowed down by indiscriminate use of nutritionally inadequate low-calorie diets, and people who can't seem to lose fat except on starvation fare. It also includes people who have difficulty shedding excess pounds because of food sensitivities and addictions and people who are often riddled with guilt at what they see as their 'lack of self-control' (these are the kind of people who sit down to have one biscuit with a cup of tea and find to their horror they have devoured the whole packet). Finally it includes people like me who, even on a very healthy diet of natural foods, still have a tendency to hold on to the fat deposits in their bodies.

A Glimpse at What's Ahead

In the pages which follow we shall be looking closely at biogenics and at how you can make it work for you to shed unwanted fat forever without ever counting a calorie. In the process we shall need to investigate why low-calorie slimming simply doesn't work for long-term weight-loss, to look at the mysteries of digestion and fat metabolism and to explore the relationship between toxicity and the laying down of fat in your body from within. We shall also have to investigate the importance of water – not the kind which pours forth from your tap but the water rich in *electrolytes* which lies locked within the fibre of the fresh fruits and vegetables we eat. This water plays an important part in biogenic slimming by enhancing cell metabolism and thereby helping to resculpt the shape of your body.

First we shall be exploring the whole question of the biological processes involved in weight-loss, not only from a biochemical point of view which deals with measuring energy units as calories but also from an *energetic* one which brings into play the findings of high-level physics as well – an approach which is starting to be known as the 'new nutrition'.

If you care nothing for understanding how and why this extraordinary biogenic system works then you can skip the explanations and turn to Chapter 18, where the guidelines for biogenic eating and living begin. But I strongly advise against this. So revolutionary is this new-yet-very-old solution to overweight that it is something which I believe needs to be understood (that is, as far as the complexities of nature have so far revealed themselves to us) in order to make the most effective use of it. For biogenics is not some list of rules to be learned by rote and then slavishly followed. Nor is it *only* a way of living which can pare away unwanted fat deposits. A biogenic lifestyle which combines nutrition and exercise has the potential to raise you to the heights of wellbeing, energy and good looks. But to do that it needs to become a lot more than a list of what to eat when and with what. It needs to become part of your thinking as well. It may even change for the better the way you look at yourself and at the world. For me it did both.

2
Lean for What?

BEFORE YOU BEGIN learning about biogenics, before you shed even the first ounce of excess fat, it's important to ask yourself one question: *Why* do I want to lose weight?

Is it because your mother, husband, lover, wife or best friend thinks you should? Is it because you have read all the scaremongering articles in the Sunday papers about how dangerous overweight is? Is it because you feel yourself to be unacceptable, unfashionable and undesirable and hope that shedding that extra 5, 15 or 65 pounds will change your whole life? Is it because, like many of us, you have been sold a bill of goods by all the glossy magazines who tote slimming as a cure-all for every social ill from marital infidelity to a poor job?

If the major reason behind your desire to become leaner is any or all of the above, although you might succeed in slimming down, you will have little chance of staying that way. For to shed excess fat permanently you need a much more *selfish* reason.

Many people make an effort to lose weight in order to please somebody else – a spouse, the doctor, a friend, the boss at work. But slimming for someone else never works for long. If you decide to grow lean it is a decision you must make for yourself and yourself alone. You may find this surprising, but for most overweight people the hardest part about shedding excess pounds is making the decision that you really want to. 'How absurd!' you may say. 'Of course I want to, otherwise I wouldn't always be going on diets and I wouldn't be bothering to read this book. If I liked being fat do you think I would be so miserable about it?' Maybe not. But stop and consider for a moment what *advantages* there might be to you in being fatter than you think you would like to be.

Fat Can be Friendly

For instance if, like me, you tend to be shy and you have grown up without a very strong feeling of your own identity, regardless of how self-assured you seem on the outside (this is something which women in particular seem to have experience of), then carrying extra fat on your body can give you a feeling of 'substance'. There is a strong sense of power which comes from having a larger-than-normal body-size.

Many of us tend to use extra weight as a way of protecting ourselves from advances from the opposite sex which we feel we would not be quite sure how to handle. Others cling to eating more than they really want or to eating the wrong kinds of food because eating has become a substitute for the satisfaction of *emotional* appetites which are not being fulfilled. In cases such as these (and many who are or have been heavy find, when they look deep inside, that most of these descriptions could have been applied at one time or another) the extra fat you are carrying around may actually be serving you rather well, whether or not you are aware of it.

Stop now and ask yourself this question: are you *sure* you really want to lose it? You may believe that you have a sincere desire to lose weight and have until now been constantly defeated by your lack of willpower or by a resistant metabolism. And you may consider yourself powerless to change anything – as numerous attempts at slimming seem to prove. But for many people it can be, not that they don't have the *power* to shed their fat, but that at least emotionally they *need* their fat. Until the particular reason for that need is faced, short of your being locked away in a prison and put on a semi-fast for the rest of your life, you have little hope of shedding excess fat permanently.

Motivation Matters

Although in recent years this fact has been much explored by psychologists working with would-be slimmers, it is something which for me never registered until I had to face it in myself.

It happened like this. In the process of researching other books I discovered that a means of bringing about permanent weight-loss existed within the tradition of European natural medicine. Naturally I was delighted because, despite my apparently buoyant health, all my life I had wanted to be two stone lighter than I was. Once I had passed my teens, however, I always refused to go on calorie-controlled diets – first because most of them tend to be nutritionally inadequate and second because I felt instinctively that overweight was primarily a symptom of less-than-optimum health and I figured I should concentrate initially on establishing a high level of health in the hope that the weight would take care of itself. So when I discovered the biogenic principles of eating and the fact that they actually work to pare away excess fat from even the most resistant bodies I was overjoyed.

I began to eat all I wanted, following biogenic principles and using careful food combining – and I watched in surprise as extra pounds fell away. But I found that as they did, although I was pleased with my leaner shape and I felt terrific, I experienced none of the elation I had expected. Instead I felt very 'unsubstantial' and rather unsettled. Soon I found myself eating many of the mis-combinations of foods which I knew had been responsible for my original weight-gain. And often this eating took place despite the fact that I was aware I was not really even hungry.

Fear of Being Lean

Why was I doing it? Why was I, unconsciously perhaps, but inexorably, sabotaging my own longing for weight-loss – a weight-loss which was so easy and left me feeling so wonderful? Some gentle probing within showed me (much to my amazement) that, like a lot of chronically overweight people, I was actually *afraid* of becoming slender. I soon realized that until I had faced that fear, and the sense of unsubstantiality which went with it, I would continue to defeat my own efforts at weight-loss.

This was quite a revelation for me. I, who like most hopeful slimmers had always believed that I lacked the strength and the willpower for weight-loss, soon realized that what I really lacked was the inner desire to shed my excess fat. I came to see that it had always given me a feeling of protection and that I was scared to give this up.

In my case it took almost a year for this to sink in and for me to decide – not just from the surface of my mind but deep in my feelings as well – to face that fear and live with that sense of unsubstantiality if necessary. Only after I had made that decision could I once again return to the biogenic principles, now willing slowly to allow the transformation of my body to take place knowing that every now and then, amid pleasure at my emerging leanness, I would need to face a little more of that insecurity which my fat had been hiding and to cope with it in new ways instead of stuffing myself with foods and food combinations which I now knew would stop the weight-loss process.

Slim for You Alone

In the past year I have spoken to a lot of dieters and read much of the literature on the psychology of weight-loss, and I have found that I am by no means unique. Many – particularly women – have had a similar experience. That is why it is so important right now, before you even begin to involve yourself in the practicalities of biogenics, that you stop and ask yourself 'What possible advantage might being over-fat have for me? Am I willing to face being *without* whatever it offers?' If the answer to the latter question is 'No' or 'Not yet', then be *kind* to yourself and, before you set out to lose your extra fat, give yourself time to look at why, at least for the moment, you may need it. A little time spent looking within can be very helpful.

So be patient with yourself and take time. For what we are talking about in this book is not some crash regime designed to hack away 5 or 50 pounds only to have it creep back on again in a few weeks. We are aiming for high-level lasting vitality and permanent leanness. This is a goal worth waiting for – if you do need to wait a little. And it is a goal which, once you decide to pursue it, you must pursue wholeheartedly for you alone. The only way you are likely to get rid of superfluous fat and keep it off is if you are doing it for *yourself*, doing it because you *care about yourself* and because you feel that you *deserve* to be free of whatever unnecessary physical and mental burdens you are carrying so you can get more out of your life and give more to your life. Sounds simple? It is. Yet very few people ever embark on a slimming programme with this clear and positive attitude, which is one of the major reasons why most attempts to pare away excess fat do not bring lasting results.

Dieting as a Way of Life

Most dieters go on and off slimming diets with the changes of the seasons – always measuring themselves against the latest tables which are supposed to determine for you exactly what your 'ideal weight' should be – and then continuing to fall short of their goals either because they can't stick to their diet or because, once the beastly pounds have been shed, they rapidly creep back onto hips and thighs and tummies.

For some, these fat deposits become like badges worn to say, 'I'm not one of the sleek selected few, I am basically "second rate".' Often there is a lot of guilt involved in shedding fat as well. And little wonder. For it is difficult not to fall prey to the multi-million-pound slimming industry and to all the seductive advertising it produces, boasting slim and beautiful women as archetypes of perfection. The media continue to promote calorie-controlled diets and 'slimming foods'. And most of us are not without at least a couple of slightly self-righteous friends who insist – no matter how subtly – that if only we (like them) exerted enough willpower we too could have the perfect lean body. The implication of course tends to be that, if only we were 'stronger', 'less neurotic', had 'more self-control', or whatever, then everything would be all right.

Such guilt is useless. It is also misplaced. The amount of fat you carry is a far more accurate representation of sluggish metabolism and of how well or how badly your body copes with wastes in your cells and tissues than it is a measure of the strength of your willpower. We'll be talking a lot more about this later.

Fat Chance with Pop Psychology

A lot of psychological rubbish is talked about fatness too. You'll find much of it cloaked under the hoary moralistic assumption that there is something fundamentally defective in the character of fat people. In fact, 'character defects' are widely believed to be responsible for fatness. We have been told over and over, for instance, that the overweight are less sexually mature than their thin brothers and sisters, that they eat out of an infantile need for love, that they are more anxious than thin people, more depressed, less happy, more neurotic and all the rest. Yet psychiatrists, psychologists and other esteemed obesity experts such as Harold Kaplan, Helen Singer

Kaplan and Albert Stunkard, who have looked in depth at the personality traits of huge numbers of overweight people, find that no specific psychological patterns can be identified as a cause of fatness. Neither do tension and anxiety, which are commonly believed to be a fundamental cause of overeating, show any significant positive correlation with obesity; in fact, according to a London study of some 700 random subjects, fatties suffer less anxiety than their normal-weight brothers and sisters. As for depression, you might be interested to know that, statistically, fat people commit suicide *less* frequently than do people who are not fat. Fat men, like fat women, tend to be less depressed than their thin colleagues.

Yes, of course there is a very small number of people who gorge themselves in an attempt to find some way of coping with inner conflict, and most of us at one time or another seek the wonderful comfort of food, but by and large fatness is *not* primarily the result of deep-seated emotional conflicts or maladaptive eating behaviours – as pop psychologists would have us believe. In fact, such notions can be decidedly unhelpful to people who genuinely want to relieve themselves of excess fat in their bodies. These are beliefs which have been fuelled by ignorance of the physiological factors which make it hard for many people to shed their fat deposits.

Banish the Guilt

Being fat is a reflection of neither character weakness nor neurotic conflict. What it is is a *biological* fact. Excess fat in the body can be brought about by many factors, such as the kind of foods you eat, your genetic tendency either to store fat or to burn it, how much or how little you exercise, how well your body's digestive and eliminative systems work, and a number of other things which we shall be looking at in some detail.

So forget the guilt right now – first because it is misplaced and second because, as long as you go on torturing yourself with self-accusations of weakness and believing that, if only you could stick it out long enough, one of those 'sure-fire low-calorie diets' would crack the problem for you, you will simply continue on the diet treadmill and you will get nowhere.

Off-again-on-again slimming practices have become a

contemporary social ritual for 'self-improvement' and 'soul purifi-
cation' (the Royal College of Physicians reported that, at any one
time, 65 per cent of Britain's women are trying to lose weight), but
hard biological facts show that for permanent weight-loss they just
don't work. Neither do appetite-suppressors, starvation regimes,
processed slimming foods or artificial sweeteners. Indeed there is
some evidence that artificial sweeteners, which so many calorie-
conscious people build into their way of life, actually *increase* the
appetite of users.

There is of course a very small number of people who, after
losing weight, are able to maintain their slimmer shape by paying
constant attention to every morsel which passes their lips. I call
them the 'chicken weighers' because most of them spend a good
part of their waking hours either totting up calories from charts or
weighing chicken portions and worrying about every ounce they eat,
day in and day out, for the rest of their lives. For them food becomes
an 'enemy' which you have to guard against every moment. But this
is a far cry from the galloping horse and from the sense of freedom
and pleasure that comes with high-level wellness and joy. These are
not people most of us would like to emulate – that is, of course,
unless you feel your personal experience of creativity happens to be
bound up with chicken portions.

The Three-Step Process

If you are fat your body is not working properly. This is true
regardless of how you got that way: whether it was eating too many
refined sugars and starches or too many over-processed or junk
foods, whether your lifestyle has been too sedentary to keep you fit
and vital, or whether there was some original biochemical im-
balance which encouraged the extra fat to creep on.

To shed that fat once and for all so you can begin to run free and
to experience aliveness to the roots of your being, you will need to
do three things. First, you will need to be absolutely sure you really
want to lose weight and for the right reasons – that is, because you
care about yourself and want that aliveness, and not because it is
somebody else's idea of good fashion or because your best friend or
husband or father or mother thinks you should. Second, you need
to gain some understanding of the ways in which your body

functions and of just why and how in your overweight condition your body is not functioning as it should. Finally, you will probably have to make some alterations in the way you live and in what foods you eat, when and with what other foods. These changes will improve that functioning biologically – from the inside out. Then your excess fat will slowly and steadily melt away as your body becomes healthier, stronger and more alive. The fat you want to lose now will go – not just for this season or while you are holding your breath and 'being good' – but permanently. You will not have to count calories and nor will you ever need to pick up another slimming magazine again.

3
Calorie-Counting Doesn't Work

EVERBODY WHO'S EVER read a diet book knows that slimming is supposed to be easy. It's all figured out on a simple formula which goes something like this:

One pound of fat is equal to 3,500 calories. 'To calculate how much weight you will lose on any diet,' the slimming gurus tell us, 'you simply count the calories you consume in the form of any kind of food and subtract them from the number your body requires for energy.' (They then refer you to a weight/height chart.) 'For each 3,500 calories you save,' they go on, 'you'll be a pound lighter – in other words, if you have a daily deficit of 1,000 calories you can expect to shed about two pounds a week.'

Three False Beliefs
It looks great on paper, but for many would-be slimmers it just doesn't work. Why? Quite simply because nobody gets fat just by satisfying a big appetite. Neither do you achieve permanent leanness by counting calories. Common folklore about slimming is based on three beliefs. First is the notion that weight-loss depends on the conscious mind balancing its energy intake and expenditure; second is the belief that your body exerts no biological control over how much fat it stores; and third is the idea that calorie-consumption is the significant factor in body-weight. All three are false. They have been scientifically disproven again and again. But slimming myths die hard.

What really determines weight-loss is not some abstract formula of calorie-deprivation but how fast your body metabolizes or burns up the fat it is carrying, and this largely depends upon how much cellular energy is available for this to happen. With some people, the metabolism does slow down and 'hibernate' from any degree of overweight; with other people, it slows down *because* of overweight. Sad to tell, the fatter you are the slower that metabolic rate is likely to be on the average slimming regime: you're faced with the 'sad slow burn'. Researchers have found that some people who weigh more than 260 pounds are able to maintain their weight on as little as 1,000 calories a day. Studies also show that many fat people tend to eat no more than their thin counterparts yet are still able to maintain their fat-stores.

Moreover, when you go on a calorie-restricted diet something else bad happens: the very act of dieting tends to slow down *yet further* the rate at which you burn calories. The body of a fat dieter, unlike that of her naturally slim sister, will seek to preserve its fat simply because it is *used* to that fat. So for many gloomy and guilt-ridden slimmers the whole process becomes self-defeating. Let's look at both of these related factors in a little more detail.

The Sad Slow Burn
As a general rule, the leaner you are – the higher the ratio of lean muscle mass to fat in your body – the higher your metabolic rate. Your metabolic rate is the rate at which calories are burnt in the presence of oxygen within the cells of your body – in effect the speed at which your body ticks over. Lean people need and use more energy in the form of calories from their foods, just to keep themselves going, than fat people do. The more overweight you are, the lower your metabolic rate tends to become and the slower you burn calories. Overweight people are 'slow burners' and superb 'energy conservers'. This is true for many reasons, some of which we shall be looking at in detail later on. For one thing, while muscle tissue is highly active metabolically, fat tissue is very sluggish. As the level of fatty tissue increases in your body, and that of muscle declines – which is what happens with overweight people – so does your metabolic rate. If you are fat, you will have to burn far fewer calories per pound of body-weight than your slim friend, just to keep yourself ticking over. This is one of the reasons why some people can eat very little and still maintain their unwanted fat-stores. All this has been well corroborated scientifically. Many

studies show that, fat people who eat less than thin people can stay fat thanks to the 'slow burn'.

The Big Wind Down

The worse news is that the very act of going on a low-calorie diet slows your metabolism even further, because your body conserves energy in what it sees to be a situation of potential starvation. Research carried out since the turn of the century has confirmed this over and over again. Yet it is something diet books conveniently choose to ignore. Instead they tend to push some kind of guilt trip on slimmers, making them feel that they are lacking in willpower or perseverance if, after ten days on some 1,000-calorie regime, they end up feeling sluggish, slow, tired and dull, and break their diet in a desperate attempt to restore some sense of energy. Diet books are also very deceptive about that initial rapid weight-loss which most people experience during the first few days on a regime. They encourage you to believe that this is good evidence that the diet is working and will continue to work so long as you have the 'virtue' and 'willpower' to persevere. The truth is that what is lost from your body in the first few days is not fat but water. Once this excess water has been shed, weight-loss tends to slow down dramatically and may even stop altogether because your metabolism has been slowed by the diet and you are simply not burning fat.

Apart from the question of water-loss, there is also no guarantee that on such a diet any *further* weight you shed will be carved from your fat supplies. Many slimmers on low-carbohydrate regimes burn glycogen (a carbohydrate stored in the liver which gives you energy when you need it) only to find themselves feeling very tired indeed once the liver's supplies are depleted. All people on low-calorie regimes burn a lot of muscle, not just fat, so that even if they *are* losing weight they are depleting their bodies of protein and increasing the ratio of fat to muscle in the process. Fat tissue is very different from your muscle. It does not need oxygen, does not create movement or activity and cannot repair itself. In fact body fat is just about as close as you can get to dead flesh within a living system. There are a number of methods for measuring body composition. It is sometimes done in sports clinics by hydrostatic weighing – that is immersing your body in a large tub of water and then weighing you when you are entirely under water, for your lean body mass (LBM) is heavy and the fat on your body lighter than water. Sometimes physiologists use what is called an impedance unit where a very small current is sent through pads placed on your wrists or ankles to determine LBM to fat ratios; or sound or light waves are sent through the body.

The most common way of measuring – although not by any means the most accurate – is with skin callipers where you pinch your skin at various parts of the body then measure the thickness of the pinch and do some complex calculations. Easiest of all is to reach down and pinch your own flesh with your fingers at the area at the bottom of the ribs, on your thighs, upper arms, belly, bottom and hips. If your pinch is thicker than 1.5–2.5cm (half an inch to one inch) your LBM to fat ratio is not as good as it could be.

This brings us to the next big hurdle if you are going to lose excess fat once and for all. It's another thing most diet books never speak about. It's called the setpoint.

Maintaining the Status Quo

The latest research into why fat people tend to stay fat revolves around the discovery that each of us appears to have what is known as a *setpoint*. Your setpoint is not a fixed permanent level of fat which your body is committed to maintaining forever, but the 'normal' level of fat to which it has become accustomed. Although it may be a nuisance to slimmers, this setpoint is overall a good thing. It is part of your body's quite miraculous ability to preserve its status quo and therefore to protect its life. Whatever weight you have maintained for, say, a year or so seems to determine your setpoint. Your brain, *via* chemical messengers, appears to regulate your body's stores of fat around this setpoint. (The level of these messengers in your bloodstream is directly proportional to the amount of fat stored as well as to the level of toxins in your body.) When your fat-supply is depleted temporarily on a slimming regime and then you come off the diet, it is this setpoint mechanism which spurs the familiar rebound eating that makes you gain weight again, with the help of an enzyme called lipoprotein lipase. The level of this enzyme rises when calories are greatly restricted. As a survival reaction to protect you from starvation this enzyme encourages your body to store fat.

In effect your body is committed to maintaining the status quo and the setpoint mechanism uses whatever means are at its disposal to make your body conform to its set requirement of fat. (We'll discuss the setpoint mechanism in more detail on pages 27–8.)

One of the bad things about this (and what happens to many slimmers) is that the weight they have lost, which has been in the form of not fat but water and muscle, becomes replaced with fat during the rebound eating which follows calorie restriction – so that after several attempts to lose weight the lean body mass to fat ratio of your body can become drastically altered in favour of fat supplies. This is what can turn even relatively lightweight dieters into flabby people with unattractive shapes and contours.

To lose weight successfully and keep it off demands four things which no conventional slimming diet can offer: increasing your metabolic rate so you can burn calories; *gently* resetting your setpoint so you don't regain what has been lost; eliminating diet hunger; and ensuring that as much weight-loss as possible comes from fat-stores, not from muscle.

4
Fat Has its Reasons

THE STANDARD AND widely held view of fat stored in the body is that it is fundamentally passive. It just sits there happily conserving energy and insulating your body against cold and shock. In truth, however, fat-stores have a very active role to play – a protective role which is vital to understand if you are to get rid of them. Fat-stores gather substances which your body experiences as toxic in order to get them out of harm's way.

Poison Store

'Excess fat is nothing less than a poison depot in an over-acid organism.' These words, which were uttered almost 50 years ago by Kristine Nolfi, Danish physician and expert in healing through foods, point to a truth about fat with implications for weight control which so far have been almost completely ignored by contemporary physicians and obesity experts.

Like every doctor trained in the European tradition of natural medicine or the American tradition of natural hygiene, Nolfi was aware of the fact that laying down fat cells is your body's way of tucking away poisonous wastes or toxins which if released into the bloodstream could cause damage to health and tissue. In effect storing these toxic substances within fat cells is your body's way of protecting itself from the potential damage they can do. This is one of the major reasons why there is so much obesity in our junk-food-eating society. Junk-foods – indeed, all refined convenience foods – are not only nutritionally unable to support a high level of health, they also contain chemical colourings, preservatives, flavourings and, frequently, insecticides, all of which tend to produce large quantities of wastes or toxins in the body – quantities greater than your normal waste-elimination and detoxification channels can manage to get rid of. When people eat these foods over a period of time two things happen: subclinical nutritional deficiencies of vitamins and minerals develop, and wastes accumulate in the tissues. So can fat – as a protective method of tucking these wastes out of the way.

The Fat Accumulators

If you, like many people, were born with a tendency to conserve energy and store fat, then the toxins in your system which result either from eating polluted foods, drinking chemically contaminated water (which, unfortunately, most tap water is these days), and breathing polluted air, or are simply the natural by-products of metabolizing the less-than-wholesome foods which make up the bulk of the average western diet of manufactured foods, are going to stimulate your body's natural protective tendency to lock these wastes away by laying down fat. In effect your body will tend to manufacture fat in very large quantities, regardless of whatever valiant efforts you may make to stop it, simply so that it can cope with the wastes which it is unable to shed efficiently.

It is little wonder that excess fat deposits we carry have become so widespread in the twentieth century, when you consider the toxicity to which we are exposed, when industrial wastes fill our rivers and seas and quite literally billions of gallons of chemical solutions are poured on our crops and farmlands every year. Even the fat of Arctic seals has been shown to be permeated by chemical poisons such as DDT.

What happens to people who have inherited a propensity to store fat is that, faced with mounting toxicity, as the years pass they tend to become fatter and fatter. And if they do go on some kind of slimming regime and begin counting calories they can stay on it for only so long before their system starts to rebel in very specific biochemical ways and to trigger extreme appetite so they gain back the weight they have lost.

Much of the nervousness which conventional dieters have come to associate with weight-loss comes specifically from the presence of acidic toxins released into your bloodstream as fat is burnt.

These wastes can adversely affect your brain and your behaviour, your nervous system and your sense of wellbeing. To shed excess fat once and for all you need to eliminate these stored toxins slowly, effectively and in a way in which your system becomes neither flooded with them nor overwhelmed with acidity. Let's take a closer look at what biological functions fat performs in your system, at what physicians using natural methods for healing mean by toxins, and at how this task can be accomplished.

Fat – Not for Nought

Fat in your body is stored as either white or brown adipose tissue. If you are overweight, the vast majority of your fat-stores are white. They consist of cells containing droplets of colourless fat. The brown fat in your body is found mostly across the upper chest and back. There is considerable evidence that overweight people have significantly less brown fat than do their lean brothers and sisters and that this too contributes to why they are fat. For a high level of brown fat helps convert body fat into free energy. This conversion is governed by nervous centres in the hypothalamus – part of your mid-brain which also looks after your body's reactions to temperature-changes in the environment.

In healthy young living systems the first response to a drop in temperature is a rapid conversion of brown fat into energy. Overweight people with a lower level of brown fat deposits in their bodies tend to respond to temperature-shifts far more slowly than do lean people. And, when their body's temperature-regulating mechanisms are unable to rise to meet the challenge of temperature-drops, then metabolism – the chemical processes working at the cellular level – is slowed. Fat-burning is also dependent upon your having a good lean body mass to fat ratio. For fat-burning takes place in the *mitochondria* of muscle cells – little energy factories. The more muscle you have, the more mitochondria you have, and the more efficiently fat is burnt. The less muscle you carry, the lower will be your metabolic rate. This slowing of metabolism is a major factor underlying the inability of many people to lose weight efficiently even on low-calorie diets. It is also something the biogenic diet can help counteract.

Of course not all stored fat is bad. Indeed some fat is an absolute necessity. In moderate quantities, the fat which is stored in layers throughout your body plays important roles in maintaining health and life. It serves as insulation and as a cushion against external pressure or injury; for instance, fat on breasts helps protect the delicate mammary glands there. Its insulating properties also help us cope with the cold. That is why most people will quite naturally lay down a little extra fat for the winter when the chills of the autumn winds first strike and why in spring, when the sun begins to shine, this will, just as naturally and without effort, be shed. Fat plays an important sexual role too – particularly in women. It gives a woman's body curves and softness which from a biological and evolutionary point of view are very important as a way of attracting a mate, nurturing offspring, propagating the species. Fat-stores also provide you with potential energy for use when needed. That is why animals such as bears who hibernate lay down a lot of fat during the summer. It keeps them alive through a long, and otherwise hungry, winter. Finally, and most important in many ways, fat serves as a way for your body to neutralize poisons or toxic wastes.

This can be a source of great annoyance to women who, fat or lean, suffer from cellulite, which is nothing less than a kind of 'internal pollution' where fat, toxins and water have become blocked in a relatively static environment in certain areas of the body such as the hips and the thighs. Cellulite is a kind of fat which can seem virtually impossible to shift. Only slow and steady detoxification of the whole body – the underlying principle behind biogenic weight-loss – will do the trick.

The function of fat as a neutralizer of toxicity has been largely ignored by most weight-loss experts – at least until very recently.

Toxins Spell Trouble

According to the dictionary a toxin is 'a poison formed as a specific secretion produced in the metabolism of a vegetable or animal organism and chemically allied to proteins'. In a broader sense a toxin is any waste-product or poison which your body wants to eliminate. Or, to put it in the words of J.H. Tilden, an American doctor and member of the natural hygiene movement who became famous for his ability to heal even the most extreme obesity and the most serious cases of illness through detoxification of the body, a toxin is a by-product as constant and necessary as life itself. When the organism is normal, it is produced and eliminated as fast as produced. From the point of production to the point of elimination it is carried by the blood; hence at no time is the organism free from toxins in the blood. In a normal amount this is gently stimulating; but when the organism is enervated (either from long-term fatigue, stress or the presence of excessive toxicity) elimination is checked. Then the amount retained becomes overstimulating – toxic – ranging from a slight excess to an amount so profound as to overwhelm life. And in an attempt to prevent such toxicity from – as Tilden suggests – overwhelming life, your body gets busy manufacturing fat so that slowly but steadily as the years pass people tend to become heavier and heavier.

Way of All Fat

It is also important to know a little about how fats can be made in your body and about what happens to them there – the biochemical processes which act upon the fats in the system, some of which encourage their being stored in fat cells. Lipids, the group of substances of which fats are the most significant type, come in various forms: neutral fat or triglycerides (which is primarily what is stored in your fat cells), phospholipids, cholesterol (not a lipid but an alcohol which acts like a fat in the body) and a few other varieties of less importance. Bodily fats are composed of one or more of a mixture of organic acids called fatty acids. Except for what are known as 'essential fatty acids', such as linoleic acid, all kinds of fats can be synthesized in your body from proteins and carbohydrates in your diet. That is why a sticky bun or that hefty omelette is capable quite efficiently of turning into fat deposits on your hips and stomach.

All fats are insoluble in water. They have a tendency to form large globules which are impervious to water. To help them break down into emulsions, your liver produces bile which is stored in the gall bladder and then discharged into the small intestine when called for. Bile emulsifies fats, permitting fat globules to be dispersed as the intestine churns its contents. This makes it easier for your digestive enzymes to break down fats into fatty acids and glycerol which are absorbed into the cells of the intestine and then recombined into fat molecules. These, now microscopic, droplets of fat pass through the walls of the intestine and enter your bloodstream. They are carried to the liver and then released back into the bloodstream to give energy, or they are shunted along via the blood and lymph to your cells for building up fat-stores.

The All-Important Liver

The liver is your body's chemical factory. It carries out a myriad essential functions, from storing vitamins and metabolizing fats to destroying unwanted materials and providing enzymes for many of your body's chemical processes. One of the most important of these functions is the breaking down or metabolism of toxic wastes which enter the body through the foods you eat, the air you breathe and the water you drink as well as those formed in the normal processes of cell metabolism. Your liver has a quite phenomenal capacity to do this. But, when it is living under constant strain as a result of being asked to recycle more toxic wastes than it can manage as well as carrying out all of its other functions, it becomes 'overloaded'. It simply is no longer equal to the task. Then toxins which are fat-soluble (and a very high percentage of those found in living systems are) are simply shunted *via* the blood and lymph to be stored in your cells as fat. A liver which has become chronically overloaded as its owner continues to eat the wrong kind of foods and drink the wrong kind of drinks, or to eat and drink them in the wrong combinations, will progressively shunt greater and greater amounts of toxins towards the cells for storage. For it is there that they will remain relatively safe, at least for a while, and be less likely to cause harm.

Fat – the Perfect Storehouse

Fat cells are, of course, the perfect storehouse for toxins since they are far less metabolically active than other cells in your body. (This is also why, once fat has been stored in cells, it can be very difficult to encourage its release.) People who easily store fat, unlike their leaner cousins whose systems work more efficiently to neutralize and eliminate toxins, have systems which tend to have great difficulty dealing with these poisonous wastes. Gradually a vicious circle is created: fat-stores lower your metabolic rate, and the toxins which your system keeps producing but your liver is increasingly unable to deal with make it even more difficult for you to avoid laying down yet more fat.

The taking of oral contraceptives and a wide range of other substances, from marijuana to common prescriptive drugs including tranquillizers, can also contribute to the toxicity which forces fat deposits on those of us with a genetic tendency towards them.

Some of us try to fight it all by going on low-calorie diets. But, when we do, the toxins released from our cells as the fat contained in them is broken down put yet more strain on a liver which can no longer cope. Then without apparent warning our body rebels by insisting that we put some or all of these toxins back in our cells – and we start to lay down even more fat.

Much of the so-called 'rebound eating' which occurs among people on diets is a biological reaction created by the need to try to protect their system from the overload of toxicity that has occurred from the release of fat from cells during the dieting process. This also appears to be a central factor in the explanation of the body's setpoint and the fat-storage which it regulates.

Setpoint Goes for Safety

The notion that your body has a setpoint – a level of fat to which it has become accustomed and to which it makes great efforts to adhere – comes from an engineering concept. This setpoint mechanism, which appears to be directly related to the amount of toxicity present, seems to be very good at supervising fat-storage. It works something like this. When you go on a calorie-controlled slimming regime, the release of toxins (and probably other chemicals too) from cells storing fat sends messages to your brain 'explaining' what is happening – namely that too many acid wastes are being poured into your bloodstream. It 'asks' for things to be rectified for the safety and health of the body. In effect the fat cells seem to be demanding the return of the fat which has been taken from them and of the toxic wastes linked with it. It is your brain's task to synthesize all this chemical data which it receives from the cells, the liver and other systems of the body, and then to go about restoring it to 'normal' if your setpoint is not being adhered to as a result of a reducing diet. And this setpoint mechanism is not some esoteric cluster of cells somewhere at the base of the brain – it appears to involve many systems all over your body. When your fat levels begin to deviate from it – when the toxicity in the blood becomes too high as a result of dieting – then the brain signals for change and you produce more lipoprotein lipase, the fat-storage enzyme. You can become very 'hungry' in order to spur you on to restore lost fat to your cells as quickly as possible.

This is where binge eating comes in – with all the guilt, disappointment and misery that accompany it. Binge eating is the typical response to the kind of biochemical anguish which is being caused by your bloodstream having been flooded with more toxic wastes than it can deal with all at once. These same toxic wastes in the bloodstream – most of which are acidic in character – are also responsible for the common dieter's nervousness, which can also trigger the eating of undesirable foods in an attempt to gain comfort or a sense of relaxation. And when dieters get the typical hangovers and headaches it is simply a sign that the toxic wastes which were stored in your fat cells have now returned to the bloodstream temporarily to haunt you until they are eliminated from the body.

Exercise is one of the things which can successfully help reset your body's setpoint. That is why daily biogenic exercise, in the form of non-strenuous but aerobic rhythmic movement such as brisk walking, where your lungs are breathing deeply and your heart is working hard, forms a central part of the biogenic method for permanent fat-loss. This is true for two major reasons: first, regular biogenic exercise stimulates metabolism which in itself helps burn fat and, second, moderate aerobic exercise encourages the rapid and efficient elimination of toxicity from the system through the breath, the skin (in the form of sweat), the bowels and the kidneys. It even improves the functions of the liver – something which is absolutely central to your solving the problem of excess fat-stores in your body. (More about biogenic exercise in chapters 14 and 15.)

Energy Lost

There is something else which you should know about a body which has a high level of toxins stored in its cells. Much of the available energy in such a system tends to be channelled into trying to cope with these wastes instead of into keeping cells functioning at a high level of competence and efficiency as in a truly healthy, lean body.

In broad terms this means that you as a person are likely to experience a sense of lack of overall vitality and, over the years, to develop a tendency to become chronically fatigued or to have the feeling that you simply can't make the effort to change things for the better. If you are to achieve permanent fat-loss you are going to have to use rational and effective methods for eliminating toxic wastes from your body and then to follow a way of living afterwards which will permanently help prevent their build-up. That's where a biogenic diet which combines well-proven techniques of food combining with a high-raw way of eating rich in living foods can make all the difference.

5
Enter the Hero: Biogenics

ALTHOUGH THE BIOGENIC diet is very old as a tool for restoring harmony to the body and stimulating weight-loss, the name 'biogenics' was coined only in the 1920s – by Edmond Székely, who used biogenic principles in what he called his 'great experiment'. Székely, who had spent many years studying the health practices of the Essene sect which thrived in the Holy Land at the time of Jesus, decided to put their teachings about food into action at a simple health centre in the beautiful valley of La Puerta in California. There, at what came to be known as Rancho La Puerta, for more than 30 years he and his co-workers fed some 123,000 students and guests for varying lengths of time on carefully chosen organically grown foods and then reported on what they had observed.

To supply these thousands with foods of the quality used by the ancient Essenes, Székely had to make use of over 1,200 acres on eight farms. There he was able to grow fruits, vegetables and grains which were free of chemical influences of any kind. The results of his experiments were remarkable in terms of improving the health of his participants. Székely and his colleagues witnessed a reversal of degenerative diseases in hundreds of their guests and students. He watched as these people gained enormous inner biological resistance, shed excess weight, and began to experience a level of wellbeing and vitality which many of them had never known before. Székely also found out for himself that, although the recommended daily intake of protein at the time was between 60g and 100g a day, his lean and healthy human 'guinea pigs' living in a biogenic way thrived on a mere 30–40g a day. But this was protein of a very high quality, simply because it came mostly from uncooked and always from completely unadulterated foods. No artificial chemicals or pesticides had been sprayed onto the foods, and little damage had been done to their nutritional quality by heating or processing.

Automatic Appetite Control

Something else within the 'great experiment' is of special interest to dieters. Those participants who had suffered from excessive appetites or from difficulties in shedding excess pounds found that, as the biochemistry of their bodies rebalanced itself, both their appetites and their extra fat disappeared. This fat-loss appeared to be a natural consequence of the detoxification and of the body's rebalancing itself from within when nourished on these natural, fresh, unprocessed foods.

What Székely and his colleagues had discovered is that the human body has a remarkable ability to 'get more for less'. They found also that much of both the overeating and the unwanted weight-gain which many people experience is the result of digestive disturbances, poor feeding, and biochemical imbalances which trigger cravings, encourage the storage of excess fat, and lower metabolism. Provide such a person with a different kind of nutrition, as Székely and his colleagues did, and his or her body begins quite naturally to shift itself towards both its normal weight and its normal, healthy, way of functioning. This is a finding so revolutionary for slimming that it is little wonder it tends to put up the backs of hosts of dedicated calorie-counters and of the so-called experts who write diet books.

A New View of Food

There is something else revolutionary about biogenics: the classification system which lies at the very heart of it. This is an entirely new way of categorizing foods and considering diet – a way of looking at what we eat in order to maintain top-level health which largely eliminates the need to worry too much about calories, proteins, starches, fats and carbohydrates. For biogenics overrides the old-fashioned notion that a healthy meal consists of 'meat and two veg', and classifies foods instead by their life-generating and cell-renewing capacities into *biogenic* foods, *bioactive* foods, *biostatic* foods and *biocidic* foods. Here is a brief outline of these four food categories and what they mean – not as Székely taught them (he did not approve of flesh foods) yet quite close.

BIOGENIC FOODS

This category includes nuts and sprouted seeds, wholegrains and legumes (and, for that matter, *raw* eggs) – foods which have the biochemical capacity when germinated to mobilize dormant life-forces and to generate new life. These biogenic foods offer the strongest support for the regeneration of cells and tissues in your body. This is why the biogenic foods make up between 20 and 40 per cent of what you eat while shedding fat.

BIOACTIVE FOODS

Fresh fruits, vegetables and herbs. Although unlike biogenic seeds they are unable to generate a new living organism, these live foods encourage superior biological functions in the body. A diet high in bioactive foods helps strengthen oxygen transport to your cells, heightens cell respiration and increases your biological resistance to illness and degeneration. Like the biogenic foods, the bioactives accelerate cell renewal and can bring about more efficient metabolic action which stimulates your body's natural healing processes. The fruit members of the bioactive group are also powerful detoxifiers and as such essential to achieving permanent fat-loss. These bioactive foods should make up between 35 and 50 per cent of what you eat while slimming.

BIOSTATIC FOODS

Natural unprocessed healthfoods such as cereals and breads made from wholegrains, low-fat dairy products, free-range eggs, cooked vegetables and beans, free-range chicken, game and shellfish. These delicious foods contribute energy, bulk, warmth and richness to the diet. But they have little to offer in terms of eliminating toxicity from your system. Neither are they rich in the subtle life energies which help heighten metabolism and restore balance to an overwrought body. Therefore not more than 25 per cent of your foods should come from the biostatic category while you are shedding fat from your body.

BIOCIDIC FOODS

The word 'biocidic' means 'life-destroying'. In any but the minutest quantities biocidic foods are ultimately life-degenerating. Unfortunately they include much of what makes up the average western fare, including: any sugar, whatever refinement, unless in plant tissue, white flour and all products made from them; convenience foods, domestic meats and factory farmed chickens which are fed on substances containing growth hormones, antibiotics and other chemicals; fatty dairy products; foods or drinks with chemical flavourings; heavily salted snack foods such as crisps and peanuts; and any other foods which either are not fresh or have been highly processed. Such foods increase toxicity in your body and tend to interfere with healthy metabolism. Therefore they need to be *completely avoided* while you are shedding fat.

This new way of looking at the foods you choose to eat is very important to grasp if you are to make good use of biogenic principles to set yourself free of the burden of excess fat forever. Let's look more closely at what it all means.

Living Foods

The ancient Essenes ate primarily what they called 'living foods' – biogenic foods. The basis of the biogenic way of eating consists of simple food combining, together with choosing most of your foods from those in nature which have the biochemical capacity, when they are germinated, to mobilize dormant forces and generate new life. These foods – such as seeds, wholegrains and legumes (especially when grown naturally without the aid of pesticides and chemical fertilizers) – appear to have a special quality of generative energy which cannot be measured by chemical means, simply because it is not a chemical phenomenon. This is why an awareness of the power of biogenics to transform life, health and good looks, tends to lie outside the realm of classic nutrition and biochemistry, and why as a result the subject has been less well investigated by scientists interested in quantifying the actions of food upon living systems than have the chemical characteristics of, say, proteins, carbohydrates and fats, with vitamins and minerals.

But the health-enhancing properties of biogenic and bioactive foods, particularly when they are eaten in their sprouted or 'live' state, have long been tested and eulogized by many highly respected European and American physicians – from Max Bircher-Benner in Switzerland and Max Gerson in Germany to Henry Lindlahr and J.H. Tilden in the United States and Britain's Sir Robert McCarrison.

Now, thanks to recent research into the electromagnetic properties of living plant cells, we are beginning to gain an understanding of *why* living foods can be so beneficial for enhancing health and encouraging natural weight-loss (see Chapter 6). But for literally centuries the practical experience of doctors and other health practitioners who have used them as tools for healing has confirmed that a way of eating which is high in sprouted seeds, grains and legumes (the biogenic foods) and fresh fruits and vegetables (the bioactive foods) does indeed encourage the regeneration of cells and hormones in the body and help restore flagging enzyme systems whose debility promotes excess fat deposits, overweight, food allergies and compulsive eating. The biogenic way of eating encourages the biochemical functions in your body to return to normal. Eating mostly biogenic and bioactive foods also fosters a high level of health and good looks. That is why, depending upon how rapidly you want to lose weight – and there are strong indications that you should not lose weight at a rate faster than two pounds a week if you intend to keep it off permanently – biogenic and bioactive foods between them should form about 75 per cent of your diet.

Meet the Bioactives

Although they do not have the life-generating capacities of the seeds and grains and legumes (which when kept moist and warm will actually bring forth a new plant) the second category of foods – the *bioactive* foods – are almost as important to anyone wanting to shed extra pounds permanently and to make the most of his or her capacity for high-level health and good looks. These are the fresh fruits and vegetables – most of them eaten raw since this preserves the highest level of their life energies as well as of essential nutrients in them.

Such foods are known as 'bioactive' for several reasons. First, thanks to the enzymes they contain (and provided they are well chewed), these foods are able to synthesize entirely new health-giving compounds in the mouth (more about this in Chapter 8). Also fresh vegetables and fruits are excellent detoxifiers of the system. They encourage stored wastes in the body to be drawn out of the tissues into the lymph vessels and bloodstream for elimination from the body. Thanks to their high enzyme and fibre content, these foods are also excellent helpers for improving poorly functioning digestive processes. Finally, like the biogenic sprouted seeds, grains and legumes, bioactive foods help heighten cell metabolism – one of the most important factors in shifting unwelcome fat-stores. The bioactive foods can strengthen oxygen transport for energy burning, improve cell respiration, lend good support to immune functions, accelerate cell renewal and, as a result of encouraging more efficient metabolism, stimulate the self-healing processes on which permanent weight-loss depends.

Food for Life

When the majority of your foods are taken fresh from the biogenic and bioactive categories you get a number of other bonuses for weight-loss. For example, you benefit from the living enzymes which these foods contain – enzymes which are destroyed when foods are cooked.

Orthodox nutrition, restricted to its biochemical parameters, has assumed that the enzymes in fresh living foods cannot aid the digestion and act to enhance the health of the person eating them since being long-chain proteins they would appear to be broken down before they ever reach the stomach and intestines. But research has shown quite clearly that many long-chain proteins such as these can and do stay intact through the digestive system. They can even penetrate the intestinal mucosae and be drawn through into the bloodstream. And, as the German scientist Kaspar Tropp in Würzburg and others discovered in extensive tests many years ago, between 60 and 80 per cent of food enzymes can actually survive intact to reach the colon, where they encourage the development of intestinal flora which produce many of the B-complex vitamins – essential in helping the slimmer fight stress and fatigue and in keeping you cheerful throughout the process.

Protection from Storing Wastes and Fat

By making living foods the largest part of your diet you not only help protect against the destruction of food enzymes which takes place when you cook and process food, you also protect against the deterioration of certain amino acids (such as lysine) which can occur when protein-rich foods are cooked. And you avoid taking in toxic substances created as a result of heating: these can range from the carcinogenic (cancer-causing) compounds formed when meat is browned to the trans fatty acids created when foods are fried. In short, you help protect your body from the further build-up of toxic wastes which work against fat-loss.

Your fat cells are the primary storehouses for toxic wastes in the body, and tucking them away in fat cells is your body's way of clearing the bloodstream of unwanted poisons too abundant for it to eliminate efficiently all at once. So a biogenic way of eating, which encourages the release of stored wastes from your tissues and from the body as a whole and which helps protect you against the build-up of new wastes, is little short of revolutionary in what it offers for weight-loss. Biogenics is particularly important for women whose bodies have become highly resistant to shedding fat even on low-calorie regimes as well as for women who, although they are not too fat, are prone to the build-up of internal pollution which creates lumps and bumps on thighs and hips.

Go for the Water Margin

We are part of a living planet, the Earth, whose surface is over 70 per cent water-covered. The tissues of the human body itself are also more than 70 per cent water. To help restore true biochemical balance and metabolic functioning to a body which has become burdened with fat it is important to consume a diet which has a high water content.

Fresh uncooked fruits and vegetables and sprouted seeds, grains and legumes are high in a special kind of water – the water naturally found in living cells. Such water is invaluable in transporting nutrients to all of your body's cells and in removing toxic wastes from them. It is quite unlike the water which pours forth from your tap, for it is a carrier of electrolytes, vitamins, organic minerals, proteins, enzymes, amino acids, carbohydrates, natural sugars, fatty acids, and other nutrients which are vital in the restoration of high-level functioning to the body and which make heightened cell metabolism and fat burning possible. It is important on the biogenic diet that at least 70 per cent of the foods you eat while you are shedding excess fat are foods of high water content and not foods from which the water has been removed by drying, baking, cooking and processing.

Most of the foods people in the west eat are not high in water content or they have had their natural waters denatured and drained away by cooking – breads and pastas, meat and cheese, fried potatoes and snack foods. Such foods, even when they are whole natural foods prepared without chemical additives (and sadly few of them are), must be carefully limited in the diet of slimmers. For a major goal in the process of burning fat in your body – and keeping it off – is the elimination of wastes from cells. Only high-water-content foods such as fresh raw fruits and vegetables tend to do this.

Avoid Low-Water Foods

Low-water-content foods act differently on your body. When a food's natural water content is removed by cooking or processing, the food changes considerably in the way it acts upon the body. Such foods tend to clog your body's systems for waste elimination and to make you feel heavy and lethargic. Both can be major impediments to weight-loss. Low-water-content foods also increase cravings for more food and force you to exert the most phenomenal willpower to keep from eating too much. Such will-power can be sustained only for limited periods, which is why so many people are off-again-on-again when it comes to weight-loss diets.

These are the main reasons why it is important both bio-chemically and psychologically to restrict the low-water-content foods you eat to no more than 20 to 25 per cent of your diet while your body is burning excess fat. Later, when you have shed your fat and when your metabolism is working in top form, you can incorporate more low-water-content foods into your diet (provided of course you choose the most wholesome of those available) but for now steer clear of most of them.

And what about that old adage about drinking eight glasses of water a day? The reason for it is quite specifically to help compensate for the water-loss which occurs in the preparation of the concentrated cooked and processed foods which most people eat most of the time. When more than 70 per cent of your foods have high water content and are eaten in their natural fresh state, you don't need to drink so much water. However water acts as a natural appetite suppressant. It also helps cleanse your body of wastes, so drink as much as you like, provided of course you are not suffering from a kidney disease or other medical condition which precludes it. And know that the clogging process which has contributed to the build-up of fat in your body and to the lowering of cell metabolism that accompanies it is steadily becoming a thing of the past.

The Biostatic Energy Foods

The very best of the low-water-content foods are biostatic. They include the natural foods such as wholegrains and cooked vegetables and legumes, cooked eggs, dairy products, fresh fish, poultry and game. Although they offer little extra in the way of heightening cell vitality or detoxifying the body for fat-loss, these foods are both delicious and satisfying to the palate. They are also good wholesome sources of sustained energy. They are the foods which athletes or people doing hard physical work will want to eat enough of – particularly the grains. They make a rich and delicious contrast to the lighter, finer taste and feel of the biogenic and bioactive living foods. Biostatic foods will form the other 25 per cent of your biogenic diet while you are slimming. Once you have lost the extra fat you want to shed, you may increase your intake of them to 50 per cent or more if you like. Many people who have experimented with biogenic principles, however, find that keeping the biostatic foods in their diet to about 30 to 40 per cent of their total foods makes them feel and look better than ever before and so they choose to stick to this proportion permanently.

Avoid Biocidics

Biocidic or health-destroying foods are those which, if taken in too great a quantity, undermine health, distort biochemical balance in the body and foster degeneration and illness. The list of foods with biocidic or health-destroying tendencies is a long one and getting longer every day as scientists discover new ways in which the chemical additives in the growing number of convenience foods, and the hormones and drugs given to the animals from which much of our meats are taken, pose threats to human health. The biocidics include foods which have been fragmented and excessively processed to alter their natural state, foods whose vital nutrients have been destroyed by processing, foods containing potentially harmful additives such as artificial colourings and flavourings. To this list belong the white breads, sugars, prepared convenience foods, most meats, sweets, coffee and all the rest. The slimmer should avoid these foods, not only because they tend to put a damper on the cellular life processes which are so important in heightening metabolism and burning stored fat, but also because they are the most polluting of all foods.

Convenience Foods and Slow Poisoning

Eminent scientists such as Canadian biochemist Ross Hume Hall and geneticists Joshua Lederberg and Bruce Ames from California issue sharp warnings that not just our bodies but also our pool of genes are being poisoned by the indiscriminate use of additives and the eating of highly processed foods which contain them. Food additives vary tremendously in character, from diethylstilboestrol (DES), a synthetic female hormone used to stimulate cattle growth by 15 per cent and efficiency of feed by 12 per cent, to butylated hydroxyanisole (BHA), an anti-oxidant which retards or prevents rancidity and flavour deterioration in many packaged foods. Then there are glyceryl monostearate, an emulsifying agent derived from partial decomposition of fats which is used in making ice-cream, and a wide variety of artificial colouring compounds many of which have been recently implicated in hyperactivity in children.

There are three measurable threats to health associated with food additives in general:

- carcinogenicity – the danger of producing cancer
- teratogenicity – the danger of harming the foetus in the womb

- mutagenicity – the danger of producing changes in the gene pattern, which can then be transferred to future generations

To the would-be slimmer there is also another important danger – increased internal pollution and toxicity.

And it is not just the packaged supermarket foods which can cause problems either. Our animal food too is laced with antibiotics on which the agricultural community now spends scores of millions a year. These drugs are given to retard meat spoilage; they are also given to suppress evidence of disease in animals raised under adverse circumstances and therefore prone to illness. They offer no nutritional benefits. Foods containing such additives fall into the biocidic category. They form no part of the biogenic approach to fat-loss and high-level health.

How About Meat?

On the biogenic diet it is not necessary to eat flesh foods. You can get the full complement of protein and all the other essential nutrients you need on completely vegetarian fare. If, however, you prefer to eat flesh foods, then make sure they come from animals which have not been raised with chemicals, drugs and hormones. This means leaving aside the traditional steak and other meat dishes and opting instead for fish, game and free-range chicken. The quality of these more naturally raised animal foods is far superior to most meats, not only because they are relatively chemical-free but also because even the structure of the fat they contain is superior. They also contain far *less* fat in relation to protein than do beef, pork and lamb.

Artificial Foods Won't Do

The industrially prepared foods into which additives are put have been literally taken apart and put back together again. High-technology food-production works something like this. In order to produce great varieties of palatable foods you first have to reduce foodstuffs to simple, easily regulated substances which will lend themselves to whatever manipulations you want to perform on them. Whole soya beans, for example, which have a protein content as valuable as that of meat since it offers all the essential amino acids, are broken down chemically so this protein can be extracted. It will then readily accept dyes and flavourings. Its texture is altered by more processing and eventually it becomes the ersatz meat now being fed to the British public. But this is certainly not the same protein which was originally found in the soya beans. The act of processing itself has altered it and destroyed important information necessary to the living body if it is to live at a high level of wellbeing. In the words of Ross Hume Hall, 'The produce contains the same number of calories as the original soya protein, but it now consists of a set of naked molecules completely divorced from any natural context.' In effect it has become a totally fabricated product – a biocidic food – something which has no place on the table of the biogenic slimmer. Eating biocidic foods in quantity brings toxic wastes into your body and creates by-products of metabolism which spur the laying down of yet more fat. Afterwards, if you care about maintaining your new leanness and vitality they should be eaten only very occasionally and in very small quantities.

Enough said about what to avoid. Now let's take a closer look at some of the extraordinarily beneficial ways in which living foods can affect the body.

6
The Light of Metabolism

THE IDEA THAT living foods – particularly the biogenic foods – have special properties for both weight-loss and high-level health is mind-blowing for most people. For we have been brought up to consider food only in terms of categories such as protein, carbohydrate, fats and fibre and to measure energy only in terms of calories. So before we investigate more deeply some of the quite remarkable effects of the biogenic diet on weight-loss, overall health and good looks, let's take a look at just what is so special about living foods.

Fresh fruits and vegetables and sprouted seeds and grains and pulses have the highest complement of vitamins and minerals, essential fatty acids, easily assimilated top-quality protein, fibre and wholesome carbohydrate found in nature. Such undegraded natural tissues supply your body with the substances it needs for its metabolic biochemical reactions to function at a high level of efficiency. This is exactly what you want to encourage – steady and permanent fat-loss in an overweight body whose metabolism has become sluggish and inefficient as a result of lowered vitality and subclinical nutritional deficiencies from having lived on a less-than-optimal diet over a period of years.

The Secrets of Lean Vitality
A lean and healthy human body remains that way thanks to an exquisitely ordered collection of biochemical events. These events are highly dependent on the body having available to it all of the nutritional substances it needs and on its not being overloaded with the burdens of excess toxicity which can come from overeating,

from eating the wrong kinds of foods or foods in the wrong combinations, from taking too much alcohol or drugs or from living in a polluted environment.

When supplied with oxygen, water, fuel and all the essential nutrients they require, your cells can carry out the work of keeping you alive, healthy and beautiful with superb efficiency. This work is called *metabolism* – the sum total of all the chemical and physical changes in the body which make you able to live. Metabolism involves a lot of different processes such as the burning of fuel to make energy, the building up of new living materials from nutritional substances and the breakdown of old materials in your tissues which have outlived their usefulness.

As we've seen, the efficiency with which metabolism takes place in your body – the rate at which you burn energy – determines how easily you gain and lose weight. If your metabolic processes are sluggish then you will tend to become heavy and to hold on to your fat. If they are efficient, you will tend to be one of those people who can eat as much as they like and stay slim. Because of the remarkable nutrient potency of the living foods which form three-quarters of the biogenic diet, and because of other more subtle qualities of living foods which we will be examining soon, such a way of eating not only triggers efficient elimination of even long-standing stored wastes from the body, it also heightens metabolic processes on which the burning of the fat stored in your cells depends.

Tiny Chemical Factories
This burning of energy takes place within cells. Each cell is made up of many billions of molecules. These include protein molecules, which are the largest, and all the biological chemicals from vitamins and minerals to special *metabolites* made from them which make possible growth and life. Each cell behaves like a tiny chemical-cum-energy factory in which all these different kinds of molecules are arranged in an ordered manner to create the 'machinery' of metabolism. In these living cells you will find no nuts and bolts, no wheels, spindles or gears, yet the machinery built from these various molecules – *via* the various metabolic pathways for biochemical transformations – is so perfectly structured that every

kind of cell in the human body should be able to carry out the specific work needed from it.

In a lean and healthy person this metabolic machinery operates well. Energy to make the cell go is constantly being gleaned from the burning of fuel. And a very mysterious kind of burning it is, because, unlike the fire in a furnace and unlike the kind of chemical burning carried out in laboratories, it takes place at body temperature and needs no strong alkalis or acids to make it happen. The secret of this mysterious burning lies in one word: enzymes.

Enzymes – Keys to Life

Enzymes are a special brand of protein molecules which, simply by being present, cause chemical changes to take place. They are actually proteins which have been built by living cells – another miracle of nature.

Literally thousands of enzymes are known in the body, each one having a specific task to perform in metabolism. Some enzymes can speed up the rate of the chemical reactions of metabolism tremendously, and in this way act as lubricants to your cells' metabolic machinery. One tiny enzyme molecule can act on literally millions of other molecules, one after another, in rapid succession.

Each enzyme in your body is made up of a protein molecule which has been wound up in a very peculiar way so that it has on its surface an active 'hot spot'. When this 'hot spot' comes in contact with the molecule of the particular chemical which it is supposed to influence, that molecule becomes 'disjointed' and biochemical changes to it take place very rapidly along certain metabolic pathways.

To restore normal metabolism and to encourage a return to normal weight, enzymes must be present in adequate quantities. The major factors in ensuring this happens are truly adequate digestion and a ready supply to the cells of optimum quantities of basic ingredients such as amino acids, vitamins and minerals from which the enzymes can be made and without which they cannot be activated. The biogenic diet plays important roles in both cases.

Energy-Burning

Living cells burn a fuel known as glucose, the simplest form of energy, which your body derives by breaking down elements from the food you eat. Glucose can either be burnt to yield energy or it can be transformed into fat and be stored in the body. When the burning of glucose takes place efficiently there is little chance of laying down excess fat-stores. The process of burning glucose for energy uses a number of enzymes. You can think of it as glucose being acted upon first by one enzyme and then another: the glucose molecule is changed by one enzyme and then this product becomes the substrate for another enzyme which in turn brings about yet another chemical change. It may sound like a laborious process but in fact it all occurs smoothly and speedily so that the glucose molecule is broken apart and the separate bits and pieces are transformed through the influence of other enzymes. The burning of glucose produces carbon dioxide and water as by-products and releases energy which we can use (just as your car uses petrol) to carry out the multitude of different chemical transformations on which life depends and which give you energy to move, talk, think, make love, run and do all the other things which human beings do.

The myriad activities of human cells – from releasing usable energy to rebuilding proteins, eliminating wastes and reproducing themselves – call for the use of thousands of specific enzymes which have been built inside your cells. Most of these contain not only an array of amino acids (which lend enzymes their protein structure) but also minerals such as calcium, magnesium, iron, copper, zinc and molybdenum. Many enzymes are associated with vitamins such as B1 (thiamine), B2 (riboflavin), B3 (niacin), B5, B6 (pyridoxine) and biotin – a few of the essential growth and maintenance chemicals. And unless the specific nutrient chemicals a particular enzyme needs are present in adequate amounts it cannot work properly, which means that energy transformations will not take place effectively.

Fat-Burning and Waste-Clearing
Many of the same nutrients needed to 'oil' the metabolic machinery on which the burning of fat and the liberation of energy depend are also involved in your body's mechanisms for neutralizing toxicity – particularly the anti-oxidant nutrients such as zinc, some of the B-complex vitamins, selenium and vitamins A, E and C. These anti-

oxidants are natural substances which help protect living systems from oxidation and from free radical damage which is the end-product of toxicity in the body. Free radicals are highly reactive atoms or molecules which have a different number of electrons than of protons. They rush about smashing into other atoms or molecules in the cells, the genetic material and other bodily tissues and can wreak havoc with metabolic functions. The majority of our degenerative diseases – as well as ageing itself – are directly related to free radical damage. This finding – still relatively new – has profound implications. If we can protect the body from the toxicity which results in free radical damage then we can go a long way towards preventing degenerative diseases and premature ageing as well as being able to encourage weight-loss.

Anti-oxidant nutrients can play an important role in fat-shedding. In fact they can be used as an entirely optional adjunct to the biogenic diet to further stimulate detoxification and to encourage the more rapid restoration of normal metabolic pathways. As such they are superlative detoxifiers.

Double-Barrelled Help

From a biochemical point of view the task which the biogenic diet performs for improving metabolism and encouraging the burning of stored fat is twofold. First, it provides the highest possible level of naturally derived nutrients which go into the metabolic enzymes or are necessary for them to do their work; and second, it diminishes the need for these nutrients to be channelled into the body's toxicity-neutralizing mechanisms, leaving them free to further support cellular metabolism and fat-burning. This is thanks to the phenomenal ability which living foods have to eliminate toxicity. It is an ability so remarkable that they have been used successfully to treat even quite serious and chronic illness – from arthritis to diabetes, high blood pressure and cancer.

The Life Energies

Actually there is more to the metabolic improvements effected by biogenic and bioactive foods than one can measure through biochemical means alone. All energy ultimately comes from the sun. It gets into our foods through the process of photosynthesis which plants carry out: they take in water and carbon dioxide and, thanks to enzymes they contain, in the presence of chlorophyll they produce carbohydrates (which we eat) and oxygen.

We get three types of energy from our food: kinetic energy for motion, electrical energy to maintain cell-wall integrity and drive muscle and nerve impulses, and chemical energy for the manufacture, storage and transport of chemicals for metabolic processes. But sunlight, through photosynthesis in plants, is the primary source of all three. This fact, although widely known and completely accepted, is too often forgotten when considering the kind of energetic information needed for high-level health which is passed on to us through the foods we eat.

The great European physician Max Bircher-Benner, who was an expert on the healing properties of fresh live foods, always insisted that, because biogenic and bioactive foods were still living, they contained a special health-enhancing quality of energy directly derived from the sun during the process of photosynthesis. When we eat these foods, he said, this special energy is passed on to us. He referred to it as 'sunlight quanta' or 'lifeforce'. By and large Bircher-Benner's assertions were pooh-poohed by scientists of his day. Now many more biochemists and nutritionists consider that there is truth in what he taught. For by no means all of the biological 'information' for health which passes to us through the foods we eat is of a *chemical* nature alone. Much research into physics and the new biology demonstrates that there are other subtle forms of energy which animate life carried in living systems, plants and animals. These subtle energies can play a central part in enhancing metabolism, rebalancing your body's functions and eliminating excess fat-stores. This is something which has been long known and much used by doctors and other health practitioners who rely on magnificently complex yet extraordinarily simple natural techniques for healing such as water therapy, breathing disciplines and diets centred on living foods. Recently, however, thanks to the work of many highly resprected scientists who have been looking both at just what kind of biological 'information' comes to us through the foods we eat and at subtle energies present in the environment in which we live – and thanks to their colleagues who have begun to measure such things as electrical fields in living cells – a great deal of strong evidence has emerged to show that the magnetic, electromagnetic, electrostatic, and other subtle energy properties of living food and of the body itself are central to how well metabolism functions and how healthy we are.

In the United States Robert O. Becker, an orthopaedic surgeon, nominated for a Nobel prize for his work on the regeneration of tissue through electromagnetic fields, has shown that electric conduction mechanisms in the body appear to form the basis of control systems in living organisms, and that the metabolic functions of living cells can be significantly influenced by electro-magnetic means. Other scientists such as F.S.C. Northrop and Harold Saxton Burr showed the presence of what they call 'life fields' or 'L-fields' around seeds. By measuring the intensity of L-fields they are able to predict how healthy or unhealthy plants grown from them will be. They have also found that, when seeds are subjected to chemicals or heated, their fields become significantly weaker – in Bircher-Benner's terms, losses in sunlight quanta or lifeforce take place.

Living Light

Very recently a highly respected German scientist, Fritz-Albert Popp, in collaboration with a team in China has shown that, just as Bircher-Benner taught, living cells of plants emit light in the form of biophoton radiation and that in the process of dying cells radiate this light very intensely. Meanwhile American cancer researcher Herbert A. Pohl has shown that living cells produce natural alternating-current (AC) fields which he believes reflect biological events necessary for cell metabolism, health and growth.

Doctors and scientists working with biogenic principles for restoring health and normal weight to their patients have long been aware that many of the reasons why living foods such as fresh raw fruits and vegetables and life-generating foods such as seeds and sprouts are so beneficial for reducing fat deposits can only begin to be explained fully once we have a better grasp of just how these subtle energies in biogenic and bioactive foods act upon our living systems – how they act to encourage detoxification, to heighten enzyme activity, to improve cellular metabolism, to encourage fat-burning and to foster the quite marvellous kind of internal living sculpture which can restore some of the most neglected of overweight bodies to their natural leaner form.

It may be years before we have a full understanding of what is going on as a person on a biogenic diet begins to reap the rewards of a slimmer, firmer body and a healthier, more energetic way of being. In fact we will probably never have the full answer, although the work of scientists such as Becker, Popp and Pohl is rapidly taking us nearer that goal. Meanwhile we can make good use of the practical principles of biogenics to gain benefits. For you don't need to understand everything about a motor car to make it go. There is a great deal which *is* known about what these simple living foods can accomplish as part of what needs to happen for excess fat to be shed and the body's metabolic processes to be normalized. And that, after all, is what we're after. Let's look at some of these things.

7
Cell Vitality Plus

AS WE'VE SEEN, a major problem in achieving successful fat-loss on a typical low-calorie slimming diet is the way in which, the more you diet, the lower your metabolism tends to get. This problem can be so bad in some slimmers that they cannot shed weight successfully even on as little as a few hundred calories a day. Studies show that such people experience a significant drop in metabolic rate within a few weeks while still remaining very much overweight.

British researcher Derek Miller of Queen Elizabeth College, London, carried out a study of 29 women who, although they were members of slimming clubs, claimed they were not able to shed weight on a calorie-restricted diet (although each of them had lost some weight in the beginning). He put these women in an isolated country house for three weeks and maintained them on a strict regime of 1,500 calories a day. Nine out of the group remained at the same weight and one actually gained a few pounds. What Miller and his colleague concluded was that it is possible to come to the limits of one's capacity for slimming. For it appears that in some people metabolic adjustments to lowered calorie intake make any further weight-loss virtually impossible.

No one knows exactly what causes the decrease in metabolic rate which underlies your body's inability to shed further fat. But one of the few things known to counteract it is exercise, which forms a very important part of the biogenic lifestyle. Another is the biogenic diet itself – a way of eating high in living foods which has the ability to improve your cells' use of oxygen, to strengthen microcirculation so that oxygen-rich blood efficiently reaches the cells that need it, to clear away impediments to the smooth running of metabolic machinery by supplying a high level of the necessary essential vitamins and minerals, and to enhance the microelectrical potentials of the cells. Together, regular biogenic exercise and the biogenic diet form an unbeatable combination for permanent fat-loss.

Bridging the Oxygen Gap

Ageing people, fat people who have a slow metabolism and people who get insufficient physical exercise have something in common: all of them tend to make poor use of oxygen on a cellular level. A major consequence of dieting related to the slowing of metabolism that prevents further weight-loss is the fact that your body has dramatically lowered its use of oxygen.

In order to achieve a healthy metabolism the energy you take in from your food needs to be in balance with the energy you take in from oxygen. The usual low-calorie slimming regime tends to decrease your body's use of oxygen at a cellular level. Counter-acting this is a two-step process. First, you need to take in more oxygen – something which occurs with regular aerobic exercise. Second, you need to enhance cellular respiration – to improve the way in which your cells make use of the oxygen available. This can be accomplished through the biogenic diet. Let's look at step one and step two a little more closely.

Oxygen-Gathering – Oxygen-Burning

Regular exercise strengthens your heart so that it is more efficient at delivering oxygenated blood to your muscles. It also heightens cellular functions in the muscles so that these cells become more efficient at extracting the oxygen which has been sent to them. A well-exercised strong heart pumps more blood with each beat. As you become fitter through aerobic exercise the number of oxygen-carrying red cells in your blood also increases. Moreover, your smaller blood vessels – the capillaries – enlarge so that more blood can flow through them. Finally, the rate at which enzymes in your muscle cells use the oxygen available to them is increased.

So much for step one. Step two is brought about by the biogenic diet, which – thanks to the large proportion of living foods it contains – can also dramatically improve the efficiency with which your cells use oxygen.

Almost 50 years ago Hans Eppinger, chief doctor at the First Medical Clinic of the University of Vienna, showed that a biogenic way of eating leads to increased cellular respiration. This it does in a number of ways by creating a kind of positive feedback loop where one cycle adds impetus to the next until cell metabolism is heightened. It eliminates accumulated wastes and toxins from cells and tissues. It supplies the level of nutrients essential for optimal cell function. And, perhaps most important of all, it heightens the microelectrical tensions associated with cell vitality so that even cells in a particularly sluggish and neglected system are revitalized. They become better able to burn calories in the presence of oxygen and to produce energy efficiently both for fat-burning and for carrying out the housekeeping on which the health of your body depends.

Microcirculation and Efficient Metabolism
Capillaries are minute blood vessels which form the vast network of microcirculation throughout your body. It is their responsibility to deliver oxygen-rich blood for it to be used by the cells. So important are these fine vessels that nature has supplied you with incredible lengths of them. If you were to attach all the capillaries in your body end to end they would measure some 60,000 miles in length – more than twice around the world. On the state of your capillaries depends to a great extent the condition of your body as a whole. And *vice versa*, for capillary state and pattern are part of your bodily condition and can be used to monitor it. Capillaries are the arbitrators of cell nutrition, respiration and elimination. It is through these capillaries that nutrients and oxygen are carried. Each of them has tiny 'pores' which allow plasma but not red blood cells to seep through and pass into the body fluid. This is how nutrients are delivered and wastes eliminated from tissues. Without a good microcirculation, metabolism cannot take place efficiently. That is why the capillaries play a vital part in the successful elimination of excess fat deposits with all their stored toxins.

Unfortunately, over the years the capillaries of people living on the average western diet, with its excessive quantities of fat, protein and refined and processed foods, can become twisted, distended and highly porous. When they do, proteins seep through and deposit themselves between the tissues and the capillary walls, where they interfere with proper oxygen exchange and impede nutrient delivery and waste elimination. This can gradually starve cells, tissues and organs of all they need to function properly and can also lower cellular metabolic activity. Such changes in microcirculation can not only lower overall vitality – since none of your body's parts are receiving the oxygen and nutrients they need for healthy metabolic functions – but also predispose you to degenerative illness and to rapid ageing. A biogenic way of eating helps restore normal microcirculation and thereby not only heightens metabolism, which is necessary for efficient fat-burning and weight-loss, but in a very real way rejuvenates your body at a cellular level.

Tensions of Vitality
The interchange of chemicals and energy between the microcirculation and the cells takes place through two thin membranes and a fine interstitial space. And it happens only because the cells and capillaries have what is known as 'selective capacity'. This means they are able to absorb the substances they need and to reject what is harmful or unnecessary for metabolic processes. This capacity is the result of antagonist chemical and microelectrical tensions in the cells and tissues of all living systems. When you die these microelectrical tensions are lost completely. When you suffer from a chronic degenerative condition or when metabolism is lowered they are drastically reduced. The stronger the tensions – the more intense these antagonisms – the healthier and more vital your body will be and the more efficiently it will be able to burn off stored fat and eliminate toxicity.

The chronic low energy and lowered metabolism which typically occur in slimmers on low-calorie regimes accompany a decrease in chemical and microelectrical tensions and a loss in selective capacity. This situation in turn leads to a lowering of cell metabolism and to a slowing down of cell reproduction. It can also result in a weakening of the capillary walls and in the gradual build-up in the interstitial spaces of a sticky 'marsh' derived from excess waste products. This marsh, or tissue sludge, impedes biochemical processes and tends to lower metabolism even further. It is the common factor both in persistent cellulite in women's bodies and in the tendency to store and to maintain a high level of fat deposits.

Eppinger and another German scientist, Karl Eimer, discovered that living foods can change all this. They claim it is because they steadily *increase* selective capacity by heightening electrical potentials between tissue cells and capillary blood. This improves the ability of your capillaries to regulate the transport of nutrients. It also helps detoxify the system, removing any sticky marsh of waste products present. A biogenic way of eating, together with regular exercise, breaks through that vicious circle of weight-loss, fat-gain and battle of the bulge, replacing it with a well-functioning metabolism which makes detoxification and fat-loss a steady, straightforward occurrence.

Doctors are Rediscovering Nature

The way in which a biogenic diet helps to heighten metabolism and stimulates detoxification – both absolutely central issues if you are to get rid of the excess fat-stores you are carrying – is to my knowledge something unique to living foods. The benefits of such a diet are by no means limited to weight-loss alone. In fact, shedding excess fat from the body is little more than a 'side-effect' of improved metabolic health overall. Very much the same diet of fresh foods is used in the natural treatment of cancer, arthritis and other chronic illnesses throughout the world.

Most of the research carried out into the effects of such a diet on health and metabolism, however, has been done abroad over a period of many years and has been published in other than English languages. Also, the clinical experience of doctors using such a diet belongs to a tradition of natural medicine which lies outside the awareness of most allopathic physicians. This is a major reason why biogenics is not more widely known. Recently, however, a growing number of doctors and health practitioners have begun to use diets high in living foods with their patients both for weight-loss and to encourage the healing of illness, so this is now changing rapidly. And none too soon, for the powers for enhancing energy levels, health and good looks which are implicit in a biogenic way of life are urgently needed.

8
Nature's Way to Appetite Control

PROBABLY THE WORST thing any slimmer ever has to face is the feeling of never being satisfied – living with continual hunger. So common is this (not only with overweight people but sometimes even with their slim brothers and sisters as well) that it is important to understand why it occurs and what, with the help of biogenics, can be done about it. For persistent hunger is one of the factors which prevents people on conventional slimming diets from being able to shed excess fat permanently.

Excessive hunger can have many causes, both emotional and physiological. By far the most common (and alas usually the most ignored) is chronically disturbed digestion. If you have been eating irregularly, or eating too much food, or eating foods which are too full of fat or are refined and over-processed, then your natural appetite will have become disturbed. To what extent depends both upon the kind of digestive system you have inherited and on how badly, in physiological terms, it has been abused. But almost every overweight body is a nutritionally starved body despite the number of calories it has consumed over the years. Its endocrine system, circulation, bones and nerves are under constant stress. And so is its digestive system.

Poor Nourishment Creates Hunger
The digestive system of a chronic overeater or of someone who has been living on highly processed or chemically altered foods simply cannot function normally. For it is living in a state of persistent stimulation and it experiences the constant overproduction of digestive juices. In such a case the body will not be receiving an

adequate supply of all of the vitamins and minerals needed to trigger the enzyme reactions necessary for the breakdown of foodstuffs into their essential nutrients so that they can be assimilated into the cells. This leads to deficiencies in important enzymes needed to break down your foods fully and to provide nutrients for cell use. It also leads to a slow-down in metabolic machinery. Many people in this state experience chronic hunger as a physical expression of subclinical nutritional deficiencies. The cells of their bodies are crying out for nourishment which is not being adequately supplied. And the body, in an attempt to rectify matters, seems to want to eat more and more.

The Havoc of Disturbed Digestion

In the beginning chronic overeating or eating the wrong kind of foods results in an over-acidic and irritated stomach. In time this leads to a slack, acid-poor stomach with all the chronic inflammation of the intestines and bile duct that tends to accompany this state. Such a series of events occurs in almost every case of chronic overweight, and is typical of people who suffer from food sensitivities as well.

In fact food sensitivities very often accompany overweight. Many a woman who reaches for that biscuit to go with her cup of tea and then finds herself eating the whole pack is experiencing the kind of allergy-addiction which forms the basis of food and chemical sensitivities. Such food 'allergies' contribute greatly to weight-gain not only because they stimulate many people to eat far too much – particularly of those foods to which they are sensitive – but also because eating foods to which you are sensitive produces a very high level of toxic wastes in the system – far more than your liver and your lymphatic system can efficiently detoxify. So you find the body laying down yet more fat-stores to lock these wastes out of harm's way.

Vital factors in achieving permanent fat-loss are the restoration of your digestive processes to normal and the elimination of the kind of chronic digestive irritation which leads to persistent overeating and to a myriad other problems, including excessive toxicity and impaired microcirculation, which tend to keep your metabolism low and encourage you to store a high level of fat.

Say Goodbye to Cravings

The biogenic diet is the ideal antidote. First it gradually eliminates cravings by supplying your body with all the food it needs (at least 50 essential nutrients are so far known, but living foods probably contain many more). Also, a diet high in living foods calms an irritated and overactive digestive system so that its functions tend to return to normal. Then you derive full benefit from the food you eat and you eliminate the ravenous hunger. Such a diet also detoxifies your body, encouraging it to shed accumulated deposits of acid wastes which can adversely affect the functioning of both the endocrine and nervous systems.

The result of all this is that the biogenic way of eating brings with it its own brand of natural appetite control. And on a diet of living foods the improvements which take place in digestion as well as the loss of weight itself occur steadily – quite naturally – without your having to pay attention to calories and without alerting your body's setpoint defences. Another wonderful thing about losing weight the biogenic way is that you do not end up looking drawn or flabby. Skin and muscles become firmer and the whole body undergoes a slow process of regeneration which can seem quite miraculous to someone experiencing it.

In the words of Norman Walker, American naturopathic doctor who lived in a biogenic way (he died recently at the age of 117),

> I can truthfully say that, without exception, every person I have ever known during the past thirty-five or forty years who has gone on such a programme has not only been able to overcome weight problems and ailments resulting from the neglect of the body, but has been able to prevent worse calamities even when surgery was recommended.

His comments are echoed by fellow American physician, Dr. John Douglass, Director of the Health Improvement Service at the Kaiser Permanente Medical Center in Los Angeles – a doctor who has been a tireless experimenter with raw foods for almost two decades:

> For many years I struggled with obesity and was frustrated in

treating patients because nothing ever seemed to work – not biofeedback or hypnosis or diets or anything. Then I discovered the potential of uncooked foods and found that the more uncooked foods patients used, the less they wanted to eat. These foods are more satisfying for patients and they lose weight on them.

Enzyme Power

One of the major reasons why the biogenic way of eating is so efficient at encouraging digestion to return to normal and at wiping out the awful hunger cravings is that living foods, unlike their cooked counterparts, are rich in enzymes. As we've seen, these enzymes play a vital part in the establishment of optimal digestion. Indeed, they are also able to play an essential, and as yet little recognized, role in high-level health all round. They are particularly valuable for would-be slimmers in that a good supply of enzymes from living foods not only helps detoxify the system but also helps protect you from the kind of digestive disturbances which result in the build-up of further toxicity, because these food enzymes help make the foods in which they're found largely 'self-digesting'.

Enzymes, you will remember from Chapter 6, are the essential triggers for the metabolic machinery of every living thing – from daffodils to buffaloes. These organic catalysts are complex substances which set off the chemical transformations of other materials, bringing about chemical changes but not themselves being changed in the process. Without the thousands of enzymes in each living thing there would be no life at all.

Enzymes are extraordinarily powerful. For instance, at body temperature, a tiny amount of pepsin (one of the gastric enzymes we use to digest protein) will break down the white of an egg into small-chain peptides within just a few minutes. The same process can be accomplished in a laboratory only by boiling the egg-white for 24 hours in a strong acid or alkali solution.

The Body's Own Enzymes

Remember that the body's metabolic pathways, including those on which the burning of fat and the elimination of toxicity depend, rely on a complex collection of enzymes, each of which has a specific task to perform. In a healthy body these enzymes are constantly being renewed. In the liver alone there are at work some 50,000 different enzymes on which the body's life and functions depend. They break down fats, proteins and carbohydrates into their constituent parts which can then be assimilated into the bloodstream and carried throughout to the cells. So essential is the existence of the thousands of enzymes in our bodies that when there is a slowing down in the production of them in the digestive system or poor replication of them in the cells, health suffers and the body ages rapidly.

Enzymes and 'That Fortyish Feeling'

James Batcheller Sumner, who shared a Nobel Prize in 1946 for crystallizing the first enzyme and showing it to be a protein, believed that the 'fortyish' look with its sagging skin, fat around the middle and lack of vitality was attributable to an enzyme shortage that occurs when the body is not efficiently replacing enzymes in its cells. Many highly respected age-researchers agree with him. They say that an organism grows old when enough metabolic errors accumulate to impair the synthesis of certain enzymes. The enzymes directly involved in digestion, such as those of the pancreas, are particularly important. Not only are they essential for the complete and trouble-free digestion and assimilation of your foods, so that you avoid the experience of false hunger which comes with digestive disturbance and the accompanying build-up of toxicity, but also they appear to play a vital role in preventing age-degeneration and disease. A sufficient supply of digestive enzymes appears to be a crucial factor in maintaining immunity to many degenerative diseases, including cancer.

Biogenic Enzymes and Health

Experts in the use of a high-raw diet to spur fat-loss as well as healing insist that enzymes in raw foods are important because they help *support* your body's own enzyme systems. Each food, they say, contains just the enzymes and co-factors (vitamins or minerals linked to an enzyme) needed to help break down that particular food. When we destroy these enzymes by cooking or processing our foods, our body has to make more of its own digestive enzymes in order properly to digest and assimilate them. And, unless you have inherited a particularly virile enzyme-replication system, without the enzymes from raw foods your body's own enzyme-producing abilities tend to wane, so that you make fewer and fewer enzymes as the years pass. By making certain that your body has these 'exogenous' enzymes – enzymes from *outside* the body, that is, from your foods – you can help protect yourself against food sensitivities and chronic digestive disturbances which often lead to overeating, and you make it possible for your system more efficiently and effectively to break down your foods and to extract the essential nutrients needed to restore metabolic pathways and processes to normal.

For a long time orthodox physicians and biochemists tended to dismiss such an argument, claiming that exogenous food enzymes are not necessary food ingredients. They said that enzymes are no more important than any other proteins – that they are useful only as a source of amino acids from which the body can build new proteins. And they insisted that the notion of enzymes affecting health in any way was nothing more than a fantasy of ill-informed food faddists. However, a great deal of European research (as well as some interesting new British and American investigations into the way that long-chain proteins taken in through foods can be drawn through the intestinal mucosae into the bloodstream intact) has provoked a change of attitude on this issue among scientists and practitioners.

Chewing for Health

It was professor Artturi Ilmari Virtanen, a Helsinki biochemist and Nobel Chemistry laureate, who first showed that enzymes in uncooked foods are released in the mouth when vegetables are chewed. As a result of the crushing of these foods the enzymes come in contact with their respective substrates to form entirely new, physiologically active substances. These are substances which, because of their high biological activity, can be vastly important for health. Says Virtanen:

    . . . there occur in intact plants physiologically inactive

precursors from which active substances, e.g. different flavour substances, mucous-membrane-and-gland-exciting compounds, antimicrobial and antithyroid substances etc. are formed through enzymatic reactions. The precursors and enzymes, through which they are decomposed, are separated from each other in plants so that the enzyme reactions take place first when the plants are crushed, e.g. when vegetables are eaten . . . the secondary substances are usually the most interesting ones because of their biological activity. When man eats vegetables, for instance, or the cow fodder, the precursors present in plants are decomposed by the influence of plant enzymes and the secondary substances pass into the organism. On the basis of the above, fresh and cooked vegetables differ essentially from each other.

Food Enzymes Live On

Other European studies have shown that enzymes in raw foods do indeed survive intact to reach the stomach and intestines, where they go to work for the benefit of the slimmer. Extensive tests by Kaspar Tropp in Würzburg and others have shown that the human body has a way of protecting enzymes as the food passes through the digestive tract, so that between 60 and 80 per cent of those present can reach the colon intact. There they bring about an alteration in the intestinal flora – the micro-organisms such as bacteria which live in the colon – by attracting and binding whatever oxygen is present. This obviates the *aerobic* condition which is responsible for intestinal toxaemia, which is essential to avoid if you are to achieve permanent fat-loss.

Dr. Ralph Bircher, the Swiss researcher, spent some 50 years examining the healing properties of a biogenic way of eating. He says:

. . . these enzymes perform two functions that offer a further explanation for the curative effects of raw foods. To start with, they produce, as it were, a self-digestion of the raw food within the intestinal tract thus relieving the digestive glands . . . Previously it was doubted whether the enzymes reached the colon in an efficient state. It has now been shown that

60%-80% of them arrive there unimpaired and – by oxygen fixation – establish anaerobic conditions in the intestinal tract, the medium in which the beneficial *coli* bacteria grow and multiply, and thus drive away the pathogenic ones.

Healthy Bacteria

A healthy colony of intestinal flora – that is, the right kind of bacteria and other micro-organisms in the right quantity – produces vitamin K and most of the B-complex vitamins. This can be a great boon to slimmers, for the B vitamins are extremely important in keeping your nerves intact and helping you deal with stress easily. If these helpful bacteria are destroyed as a result of long-term erratic or poor eating or the taking of antibiotics, or if they are replaced by colonies of harmful micro-organisms, then you get a condition known as *dysbacteria* or *dysbiosis*, which can be an insidious menace to health. Dysbiosis results in your immune system being suppressed and in digestive disturbances, such as wind and the formation of chemicals from bile acids in the intestines which are poisonous to your body and can lead to a high level of toxicity, which can interfere with fat-loss.

Dysbiosis can be a major factor in making weight-loss difficult in some people for other reasons too, particularly if one of the undesirable colonies present in the intestines happens to be *Candida albicans* or one of the dozens of other mycotoxin-secreting fungi which we all have within our bodies and which are widespread and culture themselves in stored grains and other foodstuffs. *Candida* is a sort of yeast-fungus. When an overgrowth of *Candida* occurs in the body in its fungal form this can result in a suppression of your immune system, making you more susceptible to illness as well as creating many symptoms of toxicity and emotional disturbance. *Candida* can also suppress thyroid functions (particularly bad news for fat-loss since the thyroid is largely responsible for regulating the rate of metabolism in the body). When *Candida* or any other kind of mycotoxin-caused dysbiosis is present and these health-damaging putrefactive micro-organisms are allowed to grow they can also produce histamine, which gives rise to allergic symptoms. They also give off large quantities of ammonia and other chemicals to irritate the lining of the intestines and pass into the bloodstream, causing toxicity of the body as a whole and predisposing you to the laying down of further fat deposits.

Biogenic Power to Shed Fat

As you can see, the whole issue of how digestion affects the build-up of fat-stores in the body and how it can be mobilized in a positive way to help you shed them is a complex one. This is because the biogenic diet, like any other natural form of treatment, does not act in one or two specific ways alone. Living foods affect your body generally *holistically* – in so many positive ways which interact and reinforce each other that it is impossible to delineate them all. In fact, it is pointless to try to do so. For, once you have launched yourself into a biogenic way of living, you will begin to realize for yourself just what all of these perhaps rather technical things mean – by experiencing them in very simple terms: more energy, and freedom from constant hunger and from fatigue. Your body will begin to undergo its own process of living sculpture – reshaping itself from within as only a truly vital and healthy body can.

9
Digestion and Energy Crisis

YOU MIGHT BE surprised to learn that your body expends more energy on the digestion of food than on any other function. This is one of the main reasons why after a substantial meal you can feel sluggish or sleepy and can experience a lowering of your vitality. What has happened is that your body has redirected some of the blood (and therefore energy) away from the other organs towards the gut, where the energy is devoted to breaking down the food you have taken in and transforming it into chemicals which can be absorbed into your bloodstream for use by your cells.

For the serious slimmer the question of how his or her energy is directed becomes a very important issue. You need an abundance of steadily available energy to carry out the vital task of detoxification on which fat-loss depends. All foods you eat should be digested as efficiently as possible, both in terms of vitality and in relation to the quantity of toxic wastes created as byproducts during the process – wastes which your body will then have to deal with later. In short, you need to become a conscientious and well-informed 'food consumer'.

The Meat-and-Two-Veg Error
The standard western meal consisting of meat-and-two-veg plus bread, potatoes and a dessert represents just about the worst way you can eat if you want to lose weight. And this has nothing to do with how high in calories it is either, for the special slimmers' low-calorie version is little better. What such a meal does is present your digestive system with the most difficult of all combinations of food for it to break down and make use of: a concentrated protein – here

in the form of meat – eaten together with a concentrated carbohydrate or starch in the form of bread and potatoes. The human body is quite simply not designed to digest more than one concentrated food in the stomach at the same time. And what is meant by 'concentrated'? Any food which does *not* come into the category of a high-water food – in other words, any food which is neither a fresh raw vegetable nor a fresh raw fruit.

The usual response to this bit of information about digestion – information which is so much a part of the natural tradition of health and healing – goes something like this: 'How ridiculous! I have been eating meat-and-two-veg for 40 years and done perfectly well on it.' Perhaps. Yet just how well is 'perfectly well'?

If they are completely honest, most people who have been living in such a way for 25 to 40 years or longer will tell you they have also suffered any number of problems, from indigestion and flatulence to persistent hunger and overweight, not to mention the more serious rheumatoid conditions and other chronic ailments which develop only very slowly over a lifetime of subjecting the digestive system to the heavy strain of having to cope with concentrated starches and proteins at the same meal.

This 'normal' way of eating has four very negative aspects to it when it comes to shedding fat. First, it puts great strain on your body's enzyme system – the system responsible for food breakdown and assimilation. Second, it makes heavy demands on available energy and vitality – energy which is very much needed to carry out the detoxification processes for fat-loss. Third, because it does not respect your body's enzyme limitations (and everyone's are different, depending on their genetic inheritance and on how nutritionally adequate was the diet both on which they were raised and on which they now live), it tends to produce excessive quantities of biochemical wastes which only further add to the toxicity which you must shed if you are to be permanently free of excess fat-stores. Finally, it does not supply a full complement of vitamins, minerals, trace elements, and essential fatty acids needed to support health as the body ages. So, while it is true that the human organism has a remarkable ability to adapt to difficult circumstances, and you may indeed have lived reasonably well on meals of concentrated starch with concentrated protein for many years, you have not lived this way without paying a price for it, even if so far you've paid that price only in the form of decreased vitality and having to carry about with you more fat than you would like to have.

To understand why concentrated proteins such as meat, fish, eggs and cheese are best not eaten with concentrated starches such as bread, pasta, rice and potatoes at the same meal, you need to know a little about how your digestion works, and about how and why, when these combinations of foods are eaten, it *doesn't* work so very well.

Matters of Digestion

As we've seen, all of the changes to foods which take place during digestion – all of the processes by which foods are broken down into their constituent chemical parts for use by the cells – occur thanks to enzymes. Each enzyme, you will recall, is a kind of physiological catalyst and is quite specific in its action. It acts on only one category of foodstuff to bring about a particular change. Unfortunately, the enzymes which act upon carbohydrates or starches do not and cannot affect proteins or fats.

In fact enzymes are even more specific than that. In the case of the digestion of food substances which are closely related – such as the complex sugars – you will find that an enzyme which acts upon one (e.g. maltose) is incapable of acting upon another (e.g. lactose). This specificity of enzymes and their actions is very important to good digestion, for during the digestive process enzymes need to act in carefully controlled steps to bring about the efficient and complete breakdown of complex foodstuffs.

For instance the enzyme pepsin carries out the first step in protein breakdown. It can *only* change proteins into polypeptides called peptones. And unless it has accomplished this action the other enzymes such as chymotrypsin and trypsin, secreted by the pancreas, and erepsin (which is actually a mixture of enzymes), secreted by the small intestine, cannot complete the process by turning the peptones into amino acids for absorption through the intestinal mucosae into the bloodstream.

If at any stage this process is not accomplished efficiently then the full breakdown of the protein food will not occur and your body will have to cope with unnecessary and unwelcome waste products. In fact, in the case of proteins, many of the food sensitivities from which people suffer – sensitivities which can lead to overeating, bingeing and the laying down of further fat-stores – can be the result of insufficient protein breakdown, with long-chain protein molecules being drawn through the gut into the bloodstream to wreak havoc with body, brain and behaviour and cause symptoms as diverse as depression, excessive fatigue, obesity and rheumatoid conditions.

When people with food sensitivities learn the art of conscientious food combining, and practise it, many of their worrying and oppressive symptoms often lift away. There is no great magic to it. They are simply eating in a way which shows respect for their enzymic limitations and as a result they are digesting their foods fully and properly – often for the first time in their lives. Such complete and efficient digestion is absolutely essential if you are permanently to rid yourself of the burden of unwanted fat.

Needed – the Perfect Environment

Not only is each enzyme specific to its task, different classes of enzymes, such as those which act to break down starchy foods and those which act to break down proteins, need different chemical environments. Enzymes for protein digestion must have an acid medium: they cannot function in an alkaline environment. That is why eating high-protein foods such as eggs or meat stimulates the body's production of hydrochloric acid which in turn acts on the substance pepsinogen, secreted by the gastric glands, to produce the enzyme pepsin for splitting these proteins. But this can take place only in a wholly acid medium. If there are any concentrated starches or sugars present, their accompanying alkalinity, which has been passed on since they began to be broken down by the saliva in the mouth, will interfere with the process. Then, as we have seen, the proteins can be incompletely and inefficiently digested.

Enzymes needed to break down the starches of bread require just the opposite – a mildly alkaline medium. They will be destroyed by even a mild acid. Starch digestion begins in the mouth, through the action of the starch-splitting enzyme ptyalin which prepares the starches for their journey into the small intestine, where their main digestion takes place. The role of ptyalin in starch digestion is extremely important: all starchy foods must be chewed thoroughly so that the saliva (which is mildly alkaline) and the ptyalin which it contains can break them down sufficiently for the small intestine to carry on the good work. If this doesn't happen then you are likely to suffer carbohydrate or starch intolerance – as many people do.

The Stomach as Meeting-Place

The stomach itself is a kind of meeting-place in which the ptyalin in saliva has a chance thoroughly to contact and work upon the starches. This takes about 30–45 minutes, and during this time, if a starch food alone has been eaten, the stomach's normal acidity stays at a low level so that there is no chance of it cancelling out or disturbing the alkaline medium needed for these starches to be made ready for intestinal digestion.

Concentrated proteins and concentrated starches require different media for complete breakdown, and when they are eaten at the same meal – for instance fish and chips or meat and potatoes – a mild – or sometimes *not* so mild – form of biochemical chaos ensues. This leads to incomplete and inefficient digestion and to fermentation. Instead of being broken down for use, these foods can putrefy and generate toxic acids which affect many people in the form of heartburn, indigestion and wind.

A Debt to Pavlov's Dogs

This was clearly demonstrated many years ago by the famous Russian scientist Ivan Pavlov. In his experiments with dogs, Pavlov showed that each food triggers a specific activity in the digestive tract. He found that starches such as potatoes or bread excite the lowest acidity in the stomach, while proteins such as minced meat produce the highest. He discovered too that, when concentrated starches and concentrated proteins are eaten together, the digestion of starches is impeded by an excess of stomach acid – so much so that, when his dogs were fed a meal containing mixtures of high protein and high starch, their foods were incompletely digested and the wrong kinds of bacteria tended to colonize the intestine. When meat-protein alone was fed to the dog, digestion took only four and a half hours, but the mixed meal took *eight* hours to leave the stomach.

In the last century the importance of conscientious food combining, as a way of encouraging natural fat-loss, as a tool for curing illness, and as a means of living at a high level of wellbeing, was made widely known by American doctor William Howard Hay. He became famous for his cures – cures which he consistently attributed not to his own skills but to the 'skills' of nature herself once one had learned to live within her laws. Food combining has also been widely taught by the natural hygienists and by that branch of the medical community working within the long tradition of nature-cure.

Public awareness of the importance of food combining has grown considerably in recent years thanks to simple guide books on the subject such as *Food Combining For Health*, by Doris Grant and Jean Joice, and Herbert Shelton's *Food Combining Made Easy*. Each natural-health tradition using food combining as a tool for high-level wellbeing and for fat-loss relies on the same basic principles, although there are often minor variations between them.

Get the Principles Right

The last thing which I would suggest anyone do is spend their time memorizing long lists of what goes with what or fretting over whether or not the salad dressing contains apple juice which may or may not go well with your poached fish. In fact, sensible food combining is not as difficult to put into practice as you might think. It is more a matter of feeling your way into a new way of thinking about your meals. Once you familiarize yourself with which foods belong in which general categories you are likely to find that it can be very simple indeed to plan your meals along conscientious combining lines. In Chapter 22 you will find a full fortnight of biogenic meals planned out for you. And on pages 136–7 you will find a reference list of foods and categories and a chart to indicate what goes best with what.

Meanwhile here are a few guidelines:

- Do not eat a concentrated starch food with a concentrated protein food at the same meal.
- Serve only one concentrated protein food or one concentrated starch food per meal.

- Leave at least four to five hours between a starch meal and a protein one.
- Eat fruit on its own or leave at least 20 to 30 minutes between a fruit appetizer and the next course of your meal.

10
Food, Sensuous Food

AMONG HIS MANY moral imperatives William Gladstone gave the following instruction to his children: 'Chew your food 32 times at least so as to give each of your 32 teeth a chance at it.' At Trinity College, Cambridge, he was once observed to chew every bite of food 75 times. The eating habits of the famous nineteenth-century statesman and his insistence on chewing food well became legendary in his own time. In the last 100 years, Gladstone's advice has penetrated deep into the consciousness of parents and pedagogues so that most of us have been raised under such directives as 'Don't wolf your food!', 'Chew, chew, chew!', and all the rest.

Since the 1950s such directives have taken on a new slant. Behavioural psychologists, who believe that banishing excess fat is primarily a matter of spending a large part of your free time writing down how, what, when and under the influence of what emotion you have eaten each morsel of food, have latched on to the notion that, if you get people to count the number of times they chew each bite to make sure that each bite is chewed at least 30 times, and you also insist that the eating utensil is put down again on the plate after each mouthful, then slimmers will eat less and lose weight. What Gladstone and these latter-day psychologists have in common is that, while in principle their suggestions are good ones both for slimming and for health, the emphasis in both cases on chewing *ad nauseam* is all wrong.

Eating is not some kind of mechanical action which needs to be carried out rigidly like some kind of strict gymnastic practice. Like making love, listening to music or gazing at the beauties of nature, the act of eating is meant to be enormously pleasurable. It is an act which involves the sensory stimuli of smell, sight, touch and taste in a way which is unequalled anywhere else in life. The only way to experience the full extent of food's hedonistic potential is, first, carefully to choose foods for their beauty and their freshness and to prepare them in ways which will enhance both, and, second, to take plenty of time to *experience* the foods you eat. That's where chewing comes in. Forget all about the counting and the moral imperatives and simply chew your foods in order to extract every last morsel of delight from their textures and flavours. This is an important part of biogenic weight-loss. In fact so important is this to the biogenic way of living that it is virtually impossible to ignore it and still receive all of the benefits for slimming, detoxification, energy-raising and good looks which biogenics has to offer.

Food as Joy

Many slimmers – the 'chicken weighers' are superb examples – spend their time adding up grams of protein and fibre and treating their body as if it were some kind of untrustworthy delinquent who needed to be kept in check all the while lest it break out and 'do something horrible'. Some slimmers are even *afraid* of their body and of their appetite – believing somehow that neither can be trusted and that both need to be ruled by the iron hand of discipline.

It may be difficult for you if you have lived like this for a long time and if you have always tended to look upon food as your enemy – an attitude which in itself can make you fat unless you are very careful about it – but it is time to lay aside all that fear and to forget the iron discipline. The foods on which the biogenic diet is based are good, wholesome, light, energizing and life-enhancing. Not only are you completely *safe* with them, but the way in which you will be combining them is likely to do more for your body in terms of heightening vitality, enhancing good looks and resculpting your body than anything you have ever experienced before.

So forget the fear and start right now, today, to *enjoy* your food – through sight and taste, texture and smell. Devise wonderful new ways of mixing herbs and spices with simple foods that can turn them into a gastronomic delight. For that's what all food should be. You will find, even after only a couple of weeks of following a biogenic way of living, that your sensitivity to good food and your appreciation of it have heightened dramatically. After a few months of this way of living you will never need to consult a chart about food combining or food value again in order to eat well and to maintain your new-found leanness: it will all happen automatically. And, as your system becomes rebalanced by nature, nutritional deficiencies will be cleared up, digestion will function more normally, and your natural tastes for good food will begin to be restored now that they are no longer being corrupted by artificial chemicals, excessive processing and adulteration. You simply will not *want* the foods which are not good for you.

Enemies Become Friends

You will find that your body and your appetite – that 'delinquent' pair which once had to be so carefully watched – have become two of your closest friends, friends which will not only share the hedonistic pleasures of food with you but in whom you will come to delight. So different is such an experience of food for most people who have lived with weight problems that it can seem hard to imagine. But it does happen. I promise. It has happened to me and to many others like me who have made use of biogenic principles and begun to benefit from them.

This is one of the major reasons why, as I said right at the beginning, biogenics is not a list of rules to be slavishly followed. Rather it is a lifestyle which needs to penetrate your consciousness as much as it does your larder. It is a way of living in which, no matter how careless you have been about yourself and your life in the past, you will learn gradually to show real kindness and respect for yourself, your body, the foods you eat, and even the environment in which you live. For it banishes once and for all a mechanical attitude to eating, to living, and to your body. In its place it brings enormous enjoyment from all three.

If from this point of view we now go back and look at Gladstone's notions about the importance of chewing (and remembering what Virtanen had to say on the subject – see pages 61–2) we begin to see them in a completely different light. One man who did this in the early part of this century was an eccentric world traveller who had a lot to teach. His name was Horace Fletcher.

Chew-Power for Slimming

Fletcher dined with princes and with paupers. He was a friend of the rich and powerful and of the most humble (he once carried out some interesting and highly successful nutritional experiments on a group of American tramps). And he was renowned for his practice of chewing food thoroughly. He discovered the importance of chewing foods until the last bit of flavour had been extracted from them through the experiments he carried out on his own overweight and ailing body. At the age of 40 he had white hair, he weighed 217 pounds (50 pounds more than he felt he should), and he suffered from incessant bouts of flu, colds and minor digestive disturbances. Life-insurance companies had turned him down as a poor risk.

Fletcher reasoned that his rapid decline and his obesity were probably the results of nutritional problems. So he began to experiment with the way he ate his foods on the notion that, although most of the digestive processes – the breakdown of proteins, fats, carbohydrates and so forth – take place deep *inside* the body and so are outside conscious control, two factors affecting that process – what foods we choose to put into our mouths and how we chew them – are our own responsibility. Perhaps, he told himself, the nutritional faults which had led to overweight and premature ageing were committed not in the dark folds and coils of his alimentary canal but *before* his foods were swallowed. Perhaps he was not carrying out his responsibility as nature required him to do.

'Head Digestion'

Fletcher began to study the mouth cavity, asking himself questions such as 'What happens there?', 'What is present there?' His answers were: taste, smell, feeling, saliva, mastication, appetite, tongue, teeth, etc. He began to explore in depth the tastes of the foods he ate. This required him to keep these foods in his mouth as long as possible. As he did so he discovered new delights of tastes. In his own words, 'Appetite assumed new leanings. Then came the vital discovery, which is this: I found that each of us has what I call a food-filter: a discriminating muscular gate located at the back of the mouth where the throat is shut off from the mouth during the process of mastication.' During the natural act of chewing, he discovered, the lips are closed and there is also a complete closure at the back part of the mouth as a result of the tongue pressing itself against the roof of the mouth. This happens while the food is being masticated, so that it can be mixed with saliva and chemically transformed from its original condition into the chemical form that makes digestion and absorption possible. Fletcher noticed that this gate 'wants' to remain tightly shut and the throat will be entirely cut off from the mouth until mastication is complete and the food has been thoroughly mixed with saliva. 'Then,' he said, 'the chewed food will be drawn up the central conduit of the tongue until it reaches the food gate and is swallowed.'

During Fletcher's time little was understood in biochemical terms about the importance of the actions of saliva for the proper digestion of starches. And it wasn't until the late 1960s that Virtanen carried out his experiments with animals which showed that the very act of chewing food breaks down food enzymes and makes possible the chemical synthesis of new health-giving substances which are then incorporated into the rest of the digestion process and into the body as a whole (see pages 61–2). Yet Fletcher sensed instinctively that there was far more to chewing than there seemed at first glance.

So he began to chew his food carefully until he extracted from it all the taste there was in it and it slipped naturally down his throat. After only five months of doing this, while eating as much as his appetite demanded, 'I found out positively in that time that I had worked out my own salvation. I had lost upwards of sixty pounds of fat: I was feeling better in all ways than I had for twenty years. My head was clear, my body felt like spring, I enjoyed walking, I had not had a single cold for five months, "that tired feeling" was gone!'

Fletcher's Five Principles
Amazed at what he had discovered, Fletcher formulated five basic guidelines about eating which are powerful aids to restoring normal weight, functioning and vitality to a body. They are worth engraving on your mind since they form an important part of biogenic slimming. Here they are:

• Wait for a true, earned appetite.

- Select from the foods available those which appeal most to appetite and in the order called for by appetite.
- Get all the good taste there is in food out of it in the mouth, and swallow only when it practically 'swallows itself'.
- Enjoy the good taste for all it is worth, and do not allow any depressing or diverting thoughts to intrude upon the ceremony.
- Wait; take and *enjoy as much as possible* what appetite approves. Nature will do the rest.

His simple – almost commonsensical – rules became famous worldwide and attracted the attention of some of Europe's and America's most highly respected scientists of the time – Sir Michael Foster, Professor of Physiology at Cambridge, Russell Chittenden, Professor of Physiology and Director of the Sheffield Scientific School at Yale, and many others. Sceptical at first, these scientists set about testing the Fletcher hypothesis both on groups of volunteers who for weeks and months followed Fletcher's guidelines and also on Fletcher himself, who had shed more than 60 pounds in weight. For what Fletcher discovered was that living by his five simple rules had given him a strength and an endurance which even in his early years had always evaded him.

The Strength of an Ox

At 58 years of age a much leaner and firmer Fletcher submitted himself to strenuous tests of physical strength under the direction of the then famous Professor Irving Fisher, at Yale. Fisher had designed an 'endurance-testing machine' which was weighted to 75 per cent of the lifting capacity of the subject – as determined by a well-known test of the day, using the 'Kellogg mercurial dynamometer'. The subject sat with this weight on one leg and was instructed to lift his foot to the beat of a metronome at the rate of one lift every two seconds.

'Be careful,' the physician performing the test told Fletcher as he began. 'For a man your age and not in training, I should not recommend trying more than 50 lifts.' After Fletcher had lifted the weight 75 times, he still felt strong and found it easy to continue. The same equipment had been tested on professional boxers, wrestlers and other athletes and the average number of lifts until then was 84, with the highest number ever achieved being 175. Fletcher lifted the thing more than 350 times before he decided to stop – 'Not because I was suffering from fatigue,' he said, 'but because the pounding of the iron collar on the muscles above my knee had made the place so pummelled very sore.' Fisher and his colleagues were amazed.

Scientists also examined his heart action, nerve functions and muscle health, and found he was in quite extraordinary health.

Fletcher's practices became widely known and he himself became the figurehead of 'Fletcherism' – a popular movement centred on the thorough chewing of foods to extract all their goodness in terms of both taste and their potential to build health and strength. Unfortunately Fletcher has been all but forgotten in the public mind and his insistence upon the importance of chewing for pleasure and health gradually became associated with those moral strictures of Gladstone which had been popular with well-starched nannies and Victorian school-teachers: people tended to miss the point of what Fletcher had taught and practised.

But in its pure form Fletcherism can be a powerful tool for weight-loss and for health for a number of important reasons. It makes it possible for many people to experience, often for the first time, the real pleasure and joy of eating fresh good foods. It encourages the full and complete digestion of whatever foods are eaten. It gives your body a chance to produce some of the important health-enhancing substances which Virtanen discovered are created when foods are well masticated. Chewing releases in full the vitality-store of the food for absorption by the brain and neighbouring endocrine glands. It may even help protect you from certain poisons that come from the spraying and chemical treatment of food during the high-technology processes whereby most of our foods are produced.

When a Poison is not a Poison

Dr. Gordon Latto is a highly respected British physician who for 60 years has used biogenic principles and living foods in the treatment of obesity as well as a number of other illnesses – both chronic and acute. He often tells a story of six prisoners of war which demonstrates how thorough chewing may even help protect your body from poisons either in foods or sprayed on them. These six men were weak and ill with what appeared to have been beriberi. Having lived in a Japanese PoW camp for many months, enduring the extreme miseries of which human beings are capable and suffering badly from malnutrition, they decided one day they would end it all by eating some berries which grew in their enclosure – berries known to be deadly poisonous. Two of them, because they had nothing whatever to do except await death, decided to have a contest to see who could chew the berries longest before swallowing. The other four simply crunched the berries between their teeth and swallowed them. The next morning these four were dead. But not only were the first two still alive the next morning, they actually felt a little better than they had. These two then repeated their experiment night after night. Finally their symptoms disappeared. Latto believes that the saliva coming in contact with the berries in the prisoners' mouths for so long had destroyed the poison and enabled the two men to get from them the minerals and vitamins their bodies needed so badly to restore their health.

Complete chewing may indeed be an excellent way of helping to protect ourselves from the chemicals with which our foods are often sprayed. Meanwhile we can turn to our advantage what *is* known by ensuring that the first three inches of our digestive canal – that part which comes under our conscious jurisdiction – is thoroughly used. In the process we will get as much enjoyment as possible from everything we choose to eat. Such a simple practice can bring rewards of leanness, good looks and vitality that will put much more complicated and expensive slimming and spa treatments to shame.

11
Biogenic Powerhouse

DESPITE ALL OUR scientific knowledge, nobody can yet explain exactly how one tiny seed is able to grow into a plant: this is part of the mystery and the power of nature. But the process is something you want to make good use of if you are to rid yourself permanently of unwanted fat. Biogenic foods are unique in nature simply because they have the potential to create new life when germinated. They fall into four categories: seeds, grains, nuts and pulses.

- *The Seeds:* pumpkin, sunflower, sesame, alfalfa, mustard, fenugreek, radish, buckwheat, etc.
- *The Grains:* wheat, rye, maize, rice, oats, millet, barley, etc.
- *The Nuts:* almonds, cashews, hazelnuts, brazil nuts, pine nuts, pecans, pistachios, walnuts, etc.
- *The Pulses:* lentils, peanuts, adzuki (aduki) beans, kidney beans, navy beans, chickpeas, blackeye peas, soya beans, lima beans, mung beans, etc.

Those foods with the greatest biogenic potential – the seeds and grains, nuts and beans – need to form a good portion – say 30 per cent – of what you eat while trimming away excess fat deposits. But they need to be chosen carefully, too, keeping in mind the high-water rule: the items in the list above are low-water in their original form as a seed/grain/nut/pulse but high-water when sprouted. For instance, while it is true that sunflower seeds are an excellent source of easily available protein, enzymes and essential fatty acids, unlike sprouted alfalfa they are also highly concentrated. This means they do not fall into the category of foods which are high-water and which must make up at least 70 per cent of what you eat while slimming. So instead of making yourself a sunflower-seed casserole and eating it with a small green salad, think instead, for the moment at least, of making a large salad rich in the biogenic sprouted seeds and grains such as mung, alfalfa, lentils, etc. Eat it sprinkled with a small quantity – say a couple of tablespoonfuls – of sunflower seeds, or with a little seed or nut cheese as a dip, or accompanied by a savoury seed or nut milk as a light dressing. Similarly, while slimming, go for the biogenic foods in sprouted form as much as you possibly can. Until you have shed your excess fat, a huge bowl of sprouted lentil salad complete with garnishes and a scrumptious dressing can be more useful than a similarly huge bowl of lentil soup.

The most potent foods you can eat for detoxification are the fresh fruits. This is why they play such an important role in the biogenic diet. But the most important foods you can eat for rebuilding your enzymic system, for stimulating cell metabolism and oxygenation and for restoring energy to a depleted system are the biogenic sprouts. That's why it is best to make one meal a day a large biogenic salad.

Sprout and Grow Lean

We have seen how your body demands a constant supply of hundreds and thousands of enzymes to carry out the demands of metabolism. These include enzymes for promoting digestion, enzymes needed for tissue growth and repair, and enzymes required for the metabolism of fats and for the thousands of other events which take place within your body. Sprouted biogenic foods are the finest source you will find anywhere of living enzymes and of the vitamins, minerals and easily assimilated amino acids needed to produce enzymes in your cells.

Cooked and most processed foods are very deficient in enzymes, for heating food much above body temperature destroys enzymes present in it. Without enzymes, no matter how great its vitamin and mineral content, no food can provide maximum nutritional benefit for weight-loss and health.

Sprouted seeds, grains and pulses contain thousands of enzymes each of which has a particular job to do within the plant. Among these are enzymes which can be of specific help to the digestive efficiency of animals and humans eating them – for instance amylase (a complex enzyme which promotes the digestion of carbohydrate foods), lipase (for fat breakdown) and protease (for protein digestion). They also contain coagulase, which assists in blood-clotting, and both emulsin and invertase, which help in sugar conversions.

A major reason why biogenic salads are so helpful for slimming is that they help break through that vicious circle of inertia which fat people tend to experience and to replace it with a sense of aliveness and energy which makes a lot of hitherto impossible things possible – like feeling positive about yourself or having enough energy to go out for long walks or jogs each day and enjoy them. Sprouted biogenic foods are able to supply enzymes, minerals and vitamins as well as subtle life energies which encourage metabolic efficiency and provide your body's metabolic pathways with the raw materials needed to function in top form. Just how is by no means completely understood. But what is known about the mysteries and magic of sprouts is enough to leave your head spinning at these little miracles of nature.

Sprout for Vitality

Clive McCay, professor of nutrition at Cornell University, once researched the sprouted soya bean and declared that he had discovered an almost perfect food:

> . . . a vegetable which will grow in any climate, will rival meat in nutritive value, will mature in three to five days, may be planted any day of the year, will require neither soil nor sunshine, will rival tomatoes in vitamin C, will be free of waste in preparation and can be cooked with little fuel . . .

Sprouted seeds and grains, which you can easily grow in your own kitchen window or warm cupboard even if you live in a small flat or single room, are the richest source of naturally occurring vitamins known. They are also the most prolific of all foods: a mere teaspoonful of alfalfa seeds will produce half a pound of sprouts. A pound of mung seeds will produce eight pounds of beansprouts.

Sprouts come in all shapes and colours from the tiny curlicue forms of green alfalfa to the round yellow spheres of chickpeas. Easy seeds/grains/pulses for sprouting include: alfalfa, mung beans, adzuki (aduki) beans, wheat, barley, fenugreek, lentils, mustard, oats, pumpkin, sesame, soya beans and sunflower.

Because they contain an excellent balance of amino acids, fatty acids and natural sugars, when various kinds of biogenic sprouts are eaten together they are capable of sustaining life on their own. They are also the cheapest form of food around – ideal for slimmers with a limited budget and a large family who need to watch their pennies but want first-class healthy nutrition for their children. One American enthusiast calculated not long ago that by eating sprouts alone you could live healthily and well on as little as 50 cents – about 30p – a day. In an age in which there is increasing worry about the negative effects of eating vegetables and fruits raised on chemically fertilized soils and treated with hormones, preservatives, insecticides and other chemicals and drugs, the home-grown-in-a-jar sprout emerges as the pristine blessing of nature's abundance – fresh, unpolluted, unsullied and ready to eat in a minute.

Sprouts Have a Long History

Far from being some newfangled invention of food faddists and quasi-hippies, biogenic sprouts have been used for almost 5,000 years as a source of high-quality food. They were mentioned in Chinese writings dated around 2939 BC. Székely found ancient documents in the Vatican Library which referred to sprouting in biblical times. Sprouted seeds were an important part of the long-lived Hunzas' diet in the Himalayas. And in the late eighteenth century Charles Curtis, a surgeon in the Royal Navy, recorded the discovery that sprouted seeds could be used to prevent scurvy – although the same seeds, ungerminated, offered nothing in the way of protection. For some rather marvellous things happen to the tiny seed when it is given water and allowed to grow.

Seed Magic

Each biogenic seed is an unopened treasure chest of nutritional energy, complete with a life force which is strong enough to produce a full-grown healthy plant. It contains proteins, fats and carbohydrates plus vitamins and minerals. But when it is soaked in water remarkable changes start to take place. Enzymes which have until then lain dormant become active, breaking down the starches into simple sugars such as glucose and fructose, splitting the long-chain protein molecules into free amino acids and decreasing the seed's content of saturated fats by turning them into free fatty acids. Whatever mucus-producing properties the legume or grain had as a seed are now drastically reduced by enzymes activated in the germinating process. In fact the activity of enzymes in any plant is never so great as when a seed sprouts. Physicians who use freshly grown sprouts as part of their healing programme claim that when they are eaten this rich activity of enzymes stimulates the body's own enzymic activities and leads to a regeneration of cells and tissues and an overall improvement in cell metabolism.

Certainly the action of the enzymes in breaking down food components produces an edible food which is far more easily accessible for bodily use. For biogenic sprouts become almost 'predigested'. They have a far higher biological efficiency when they are eaten than did the whole seeds from which they were grown. So you need to eat *less* of them – yet *more* nutrients effectively reach the bloodstream and cells. Experiments with sprouted seeds show that overall protein levels increase with germination as well. And as germination continues the relationship between essential and non-essential amino acids also changes, so that the plant becomes increasingly more valuable as a source of body protein. Researchers C.Y. Tsai and A. Dalby of the Department of Botany and Plant Pathology of Purdue University, Indiana, showed, for instance, that during the germination of maize seeds the concentration of lysine and tryptophan (two essential amino acids whose low levels in corn render it a poor-quality food for protein if it is eaten on its own) increase. They concluded that germination is a good method of converting nutritionally poor-quality plant protein to a good-quality protein for human and animal use.

Vitamins Galore
The increase in the vitamin content of germinated seeds and grains is really quite phenomenal. Dr. Paul Burkholder at Yale University

looked at the increase in the B-vitamin content of oats before and after sprouting, and discovered that their vitamin B2 content had risen by 1,300 per cent almost immediately. By the time tiny green leaves were formed it had gone up 2,000 per cent. He also found increases in biotin (50 per cent), inositol (100 per cent), pantothenic acid (200 per cent), pyridoxine (500 per cent) and folic acid (600 per cent). Another researcher, Dr. Barry Mack at the University of Pennsylvania, measured vitamin C in soya beans after 7½ hours of sprouting and found it had risen by 553 per cent. Dr. C. Bailey of the University of Minnesota found only small amounts of vitamin C in unsprouted wheat grains, but after sprouting for a few days these had increased by 600 per cent. As for the B vitamins, sprouted wheat also contains 30 per cent more B1 (thiamine), 200 per cent more B2 (riboflavin), 90 per cent more niacin, 80 per cent more pantothenic acid and 100 per cent more biotin and pyridoxine. So rich in vitamin C are soya sprouts that only a tablespoonful of them will yield half of the recommended adult daily dose.

A New-Style Kitchen Garden

You need no soil for your 'garden', you will have no problems with weeds or with slugs eating fresh crops, and sprouted seeds and grains can be grown at all seasons of the year, regardless of the weather conditions or climate.

In short, they will produce almost anywhere. They are also quick to harvest – you simply pour them from the bottle or lift them from the seed tray, rinse them and store them in your refrigerator in a plastic bag until they are needed. If you are a hill-walker or camper, you can carry (and grow) sprouted seeds and grains in your knapsack or in the pocket of a jacket. There they will remain alive and growing – powerhouses of vital nutrition – until you want to eat them. Growing them at home takes up very little time – a few minutes to rinse the growing seeds in fresh water, morning and evening if you grow them in jars and only once a day if you grow them in trays. You will have a new harvest every few days. We produce about 100 crops a year in our kitchen. The flavour of the little plants is so sweet, thanks to the conversion of starch into simple sugars, that my youngest son carries them around in his pocket to eat as snacks. I make whole salad-meals not only for myself but also for my family from nothing but various sprouts topped with a delicious avocado dressing, a seed cheese or a home-made mayonnaise.

Children are particular lovers of sprouts. They like growing them themselves and watching their daily progress. So sprouts are an excellent way of introducing kids used to baked beans and sausages to better foods. The power they offer for health-promoting and life-enhancing nutrition is unequalled anywhere – even at 10 times the price. For instance, at the University of Texas System Cancer Center, Chiu-Nan Lai and his colleagues exposed bacteria to carcinogenic (cancer-causing) chemicals in the presence of an extract taken from wheat sprouts, mung beans and lentil sprouts and found that the cancer development was 99 per cent inhibited. When they examined the wheat-sprout extract to find which was the most active factor in cancer inhibition they discovered it to be chlorophyll.

Sprouts for Good Mineral Balance and Fat Transport
The only minerals your body can properly assimilate are 'organic minerals' – that is, minerals bound to organic molecules in foods and drinks. Vegetable foods are an excellent source of organic minerals. But some of the substances in such foods (e.g. in peas and beans and some grains) contain also other factors such as phytic acid that tend to bind together with their minerals (e.g. calcium, zinc and iron) to form insoluble compounds which the body cannot properly absorb. Phytin, a magnesium-calcium salt of phytic acid, is an important ingredient in many seeds and, like phytic acid, is rich in phosphorus: it can account for as much as 80 per cent of the phosphorus content of some seeds. A. M. Maiser and A. Poljakoff-Mayber, researchers at the Hebrew University, have shown, however, that sprouting dramatically decreases the content of undesirable phosphates such as phytin in a seed, making minerals otherwise inaccessible to the body available for use. Sprouting also increases desirable phosphorus compounds such as the lecithins, phospholipids which help break up and transport fats and fatty acids in the body. Lecithins also help prevent the accumulation of too much acid or too much alkali in your blood and encourage the transport of nutrients through cell walls, in addition to being an aid

to fat metabolism. They are needed too for healthy nerves and efficient brain functions, and they promote the secretion of glandular hormones.

The Organic Question

Ideally the foods you eat on a high-raw diet should be chosen from fresh, organically grown vegetables and fruits, for these foods offer the highest complement of substances of nutritional value to an organism. But for me, as for most people, this is just not possible. I grow my own herbs and a few fruits and vegetables in my garden in the country but half of the time I live in a flat in the city and there I have little access to anything which has been organically composted.

Making at least one meal a day a biogenic salad solves, at least in part, the dilemma about organically grown foods because, since you've grown the sprouts yourself, you *know* that they haven't been subjected to any chemical treatments and, because you have used (or should have used) spring water for them, that they do not contain any undesirable minerals or other chemicals. And your biogenic salad is an excellent source of top-quality protein, essential fatty acids, and natural sugars. (For when seeds are sprouted the starch in them begins to be broken down and turned into natural sugars which are easy to assimilate and provide energy to heighten your mood.) Finally, and probably most important of all, remember that biogenic sprouts are brimming with life energy. This life energy, which is the very basis of the power which biogenics has to transform your health, your shape, your energy and your overall good looks, is as yet little understood: it is only beginning to be measured by sensitive instruments in terms of subtle electromagnetic energies. But something that can be measured and is superbly evident after a few weeks of following a biogenic lifestyle is your firmer, slimmer shape and the new lease of life which biogenics can bring you.

12
Headstart – The Applefast

ONE OF THE best ways to trigger rapid detoxification of your body and get you into the biogenic way of living is to do an applefast for a few days before you begin. Of course, no one inexperienced in the art and science of fasting should fast on water for more than a couple of days unless they are under the watchful eye of a physician who has been well trained in natural methods of healing, and *never* if they are pregnant, suffering from kidney or liver disease, or on drug therapy. But an applefast is different. In truth it is not a fast at all for you eat as much as you want – but only apples in place of your regular meals. Like the traditional water-fast, the applefast is a powerful tool for stimulating the process of detoxification on which permanent weight-loss depends. Many experts in natural healing believe that it is even better than a waterfast – for reasons we will be looking at.

Triple Power for Fat-Loss
The applefast can be used in three different ways, each of which is helpful towards your goal of shedding unwanted fat and banishing excess appetite permanently.

First, you can begin your biogenic diet with a few days on the applefast to get you off to a good start. This will spur the rapid elimination of waste, help clear away any food sensitivities which may be present as a result of improper food combining, and banish the ravages of unnatural appetite due to chronic over-stimulation of the digestive system.

Second, you can set aside one day a week for applefasting while you are following biogenic principles and conscientious food combining during the rest of the week. This once-a-week applefast is a great boost because a day or two a week on fruit alone is the best way to detoxify your body rapidly. A day a week on apples alone is also an excellent discipline. Such a practice helps us break through ingrained habit patterns which tend to make us unconscious and mechanical in the way we live and largely unaware of how we are eating.

Third, you can use the applefast whenever, for whatever reason, you have 'slipped'. For example, you may have failed to combine your foods properly yesterday, or have eaten more than you really wanted, or your system has become somewhat polluted because you were trapped in a smoke-filled room the evening before. A day of applefasting will quickly correct any digestive disturbances or internal pollution problems which have resulted and which, if left unchecked, can trigger excessive appetite. It can put you back on the track again and have you feeling great when you awaken the following morning.

I first learned about applefasting from a well-known British doctor who had been using it for almost 50 years as part of his own biogenic approach to the treatment of obesity. He calls on it both in cases of chronic serious obesity – where his patient is three, four or more stone overweight – and also for people who wish to lose less than a stone of fat in order to improve their overall health and restore their natural body condition. When I first tried it myself I was amazed to find how efficient it was at detoxifying my body, at banishing excess appetite and at making me feel centred and well while I was shedding fat.

Apples are Special

The adage that 'an apple a day keeps the doctor away' is not just an old wives' tale. The apple is quite rightly known as the 'Queen of Fruits'. In its natural whole state it supplies valuable fruit sugar and vitamins in a superb balance to ensure efficient digestion and use. Apples are richer than any other fruit in vitamin E, and also offer a good supply of biotin and folic acid – two very important B-complex vitamins which are particularly useful in encouraging fat-loss, in preserving emotional balance and in keeping your digestive system clean and functioning well. The apple is also a good source of vitamins A and C – natural anti-oxidants or detoxifiers which are essential for high-level health. In addition it supplies a dozen minerals including sulphur, potassium, iron, iodine, silicon, magnesium and calcium together with small quantities of many other vitamins and even essential amino acids.

It was the apple which first led Swiss physician Max Bircher-Benner to develop his system of treatment based on living foods. Bircher-Benner himself was ill with a liver ailment which made it virtually impossible for him to digest food. One day as he lay in his bed not even able to rise and certainly unable to eat anything, his wife, who had been peeling apples for supper and who was sitting with him, slipped a small piece of fresh raw apple between his teeth. He tasted it, and to his surprise he found he could tolerate it. Several days – and many raw apples – later, he found himself well again. He never forgot the humble apple or what it could do to detoxify the body and to help restore normal functioning to digestion, cells and the circulation. He used apples regularly in his dietary treatments of obesity and other illnesses. In fact they formed the basis of his Birchermuesli, which has become world-famous.

Even in folklore the apple has been known as a health tonic, medicine, cosmetic and bowel regulator all wrapped up in one. When eaten, it stimulates the secretion of digestive juices. It contains both malic and tartaric acids which help prevent digestive and liver troubles. Where unsweetened apple juice is the traditional drink among country people there tends to be no incidence of kidney stones. Apples also have an alkalinizing effect on the body. They stimulate the flow of saliva in the mouth and help remove debris from the teeth. And eating fresh raw apples stimulates circulation in the gums. The simple apple is traditionally used for eliminating obesity as well as in folk treatments for skin problems, bladder inflammation, anaemia, insomnia, intestinal parasites and bad breath.

One of the most important of all the apple's attributes is the fibre it contains. In addition to cellulose – which binds water and increases faecal bulk, and is the most common kind of dietary fibre – the apple is also rich in pectin, a very special sort of fibre with quite exceptional detoxifying properties. So different in texture and character is pectin from other forms of fibre that it is somewhat surprising to think that they are classified in the same group. Unlike cellulose, pectin does not bind water: indeed, it is water-soluble. It has no influence on faecal bulking but it appears to be an excellent substance for lowering cholesterol. It may also help eliminate bile acids from the intestines, thus short-circuiting the development of colon cancer and gallstones. Because of pectin's ability to bind organic materials such as bile acids, it is also useful as a natural chelating (binding) agent to take up unwanted heavy metals such as aluminium from the tissues and to eliminate them from the body; this can be very important when it comes to detoxification for weight-loss. Pectin's chelating properties also make it very influential in helping to protect your body from degeneration and premature ageing. Heavy metals are potent *cross-linkers* which can drastically interfere with brain and body. That is why, in the natural treatment of heavy-metal poisoning, pectin is usually given along with vitamin C and other natural substances as a chelating agent to remove the offending metals.

How Much? How Long?

Using the applefast as part of the biogenic approach to weight-loss is simple (although it is by no means essential to the success of biogenic fat-loss). If you are keen to get off to a good start with detoxification then set aside two or three days before the beginning of your biogenic diet for applefasting. Buy a box of apples (usually the greengrocer will give you a good discount when you buy a box at a time) or buy three or four different kinds of apples for variety to get you started.

Eat as many as you like but eat the *whole* apple including the peel, the seeds and the core and you must chew it all very well – until the last drop of flavour has been extracted from the fruit. The only part you throw away is the woody stem. Of course the apples you eat need to be fresh and eaten raw. You can munch these crisp fruits *au naturel*. You can chop them and sprinkle a little cinnamon on top; or you can even put them in the blender with spring water to make a whole apple drink. Eat apples whenever you are hungry throughout the day. While you are on an applefast is an ideal time to begin growing your sprouts ready for the preparation of biogenic dishes in two or three days' time.

How long you continue your first applefast depends upon how convenient it is for you to munch nothing but apples and on how you feel. Some doctors using biogenic methods keep slimmers on apples alone for as long as a week or 10 days at the beginning of this changeover to a biogenic lifestyle. But this depends very much on the enthusiasm of the person for the whole process and of course on their general health. Usually a couple of days is enough to give you a good start on spring-cleaning your body from within. Three days is probably as much as any healthy person should do on his or her own without being under the supervision of a doctor or other health practitioner well versed in fasting and in the use of living foods for the treatment of obesity and illness. No one who is pregnant or lactating should do an applefast (except of course at the suggestion of their doctor). Neither should anyone with a kidney, liver or heart complaint, for in such cases any sudden change of diet carries with it potential dangers to health. But if you are generally well and your doctor does not disapprove then a short applefast is a great way to clear the decks for your new way of living. When your day or two on apples alone is finished then you simply begin the next morning to apply the biogenic principles.

The Once-a-Week Treat

It really is a treat, too, as you will find after you have got into the swing of biogenics, to lay aside one day of rest from the three-meals-a-day routine and spend it applefasting. This gives your digestive system a break and helps clear your mind and encourages the breaking of old, poor eating habits. It is also an excellent tool for giving an extra push to the detoxification process for efficient fat-loss. For me applefasting is a pleasure. I have to travel quite a lot for my work and hate being faced with some of the aeroplane, hotel and restaurant food which I would otherwise be forced to eat. So instead I carry a big sack of apples with me and munch away while I am in a car or train or aeroplane. I always find it increases my energy and has me sailing through whatever I have to do. I tend to vary the day of my applefast from week to week. Most often it is Monday (I feel it's a good way to start the week) but when I have a commitment which entails a lunch or supper on a Monday I simply shift it to a day later on in the week – especially to a travel day.

The Quick Corrector

In many ways the most useful thing of all about the applefast is the way you can call on it when you most need help to get you back on the rails again. Everybody is occasionally in a situation where he or she eats something that they would really rather not have eaten. You may find that your system has been upset by some dish you were served the day before which was poorly combined or that unwise food combinations have forced the return of intense appetite which will not go away again until your digestive system is calmed and your body balanced once more. Or perhaps you have overeaten (old habits die hard and you must be patient with yourself if this does happen) or you are under heavy stress for some reason and feel you need help to smooth things over.

A day-long applefast is ideal as a 'quick corrector' in any of these situations. Spend the day munching apples and it will help set all to rights again so that when you awaken the next morning you feel more centred and more yourself and are ready to get back to your biogenic lifestyle with renewed enthusiasm and energy.

The Cleansing Crisis

Very occasionally when someone goes on an active programme of detoxification such as the biogenic diet or – even more so – the applefast, he or she has the experience of a severe headache at some time within the first three days or of feeling moody or of having an upset stomach or loose bowels. This is a sign that your body is throwing off wastes at such a pace that you are experiencing what is known in natural medicine as a *cleansing crisis*. In fact it happens to very few people. If you are one of them, be glad – even though it may be a bit of a nuisance for a few hours, it is actually a good sign. Your body is taking the opportunity you have afforded it through what you are eating (and what you are *not* eating) to get rid of a lot of debris which you need to eliminate if you are to shed unwanted fat permanently and live at a higher level of health and vitality.

If a cleansing crisis does occur, it is most likely to happen within the first day or two of applefasting. Then, take the time to relax, lie down in a darkened room if possible and be kind to yourself.

Congratulations. It is quite a feat to be ridding your body of so much old debris all at once. The cleansing crisis will pass quickly, leaving you better than ever.

People most likely to get a headache as part of a cleansing crisis are those who have been drinking several cups of coffee or tea a day. This kind of reaction is triggered by your tissues dumping a lot of stored caffeine into your bloodstream all at once in order to eliminate it from your body. The first time this happened to me I had been in Vienna for six days where everybody drinks coffee – and very *strong* coffee too – all day long. Not being much of a coffee-drinker myself (apart from a cup of bitter Turkish coffee once every six months after a Middle Eastern meal in a restaurant), while there I decided to go along with the custom. The day I left the city I got onto an aeroplane to return to London and to my usual way of eating and found I was struck down by the most appalling headache which lasted about four or five hours. It was no fun, believe me. But when it passed I was left with the most wonderful feeling of freshness and lightness – the way you feel on a beautiful summer's morning when there is a light breeze blowing. This sense of lightness is a common one for people who for the first time begin to clear their system of stored wastes. It more than makes up for the headache or tummy upset which heralded its coming.

Compress Help

Something which I learnt many years ago from a doctor who uses biogenics for weight-loss and healing (as well as other natural methods such as breathing techniques and hydrotherapy) is that, if you are experiencing any kind of cleansing crisis, you can help your body enormously by putting a simple cool compress around your middle and leaving it there as you lie down for half an hour. This can also be done when you go to bed in the evening if you prefer. You can even fall asleep with it on and simply take it off in the morning. A cool compress stimulates the flow of blood to the area of the liver and, in effect, lends it a helping hand when it is most in need of help. It is also enormously relaxing.

Tear a piece of cotton fabric (an old sheet is ideal) into a rectangular piece which is about 15 inches wide and long enough to go comfortably around the middle of your body (between your armpits and hips). Wet this compress in cold water and wring it out completely so that it is only damp. Now take a dry towel or a piece of wool or thick natural fabric which is likewise big enough to go around your middle and to overlap, so that you can pin it comfortably with a few safety pins. Spread the compress out on the outstretched towel, and lay your naked midriff on this strip and wrap around you first the compress and then the towel on top, pinning it securely. Pull your clothes or nightclothes down over the lot and pop into a warm bed for at least half an hour.

Such a compress can be helpful not only in sailing you through a cleansing crisis but also if ever you find it difficult to sleep because of worry or stress or if ever you are having to deal with the aftermath of excess alcohol.

The possibility that you will experience any sort of cleansing crisis is slim. Most people simply detoxify without any outward signs of difficulty. Those who do get headaches or intestinal upsets in the process usually fall into one of two categories: either they have quite exceptional vitality which makes them highly reactive to change of any kind (this will mean that they reap the benefits of biogenic weight-loss long before the rest of us, by the way) or they may suffer from food sensitivities or allergies which have been masked by the manner in which they have been previously eating and which are now being unmasked by the detoxification programme. If this is the case, as the sensitivities clear you are likely to feel that a great burden is being lifted from you. In fact, the biogenic lifestyle – the diet coupled with biogenic exercise – can do more to help clear up even long-standing food sensitivities than any other single natural technique.

The applefast, as we have noted, is entirely optional to the whole process of biogenic weight-control. But for me, practised one day a week, it has become a source of pleasure and energy which I would never want to be without.

13
Supplementary Benefits

THANKS TO THE fact that bioactive and especially biogenic foods are so high in essential vitamins and minerals, and to the way biogenics removes the burden of toxicity from your system, the biogenic diet is able to restore biochemical balance and to correct nutritional deficiencies which have developed through being overweight and eating the wrong kinds of foods in the past. This it will do slowly and steadily. As it does so, your metabolic pathways – the 'machinery of metabolism' – will become 'well-oiled' so that they work better and better. Your ability to use oxygen on a cellular level will improve. And your overall vitality will steadily increase as your system becomes healthier and healthier. A biogenic way of eating enhances your overall nutritional status, the functioning of your immune system, your mental and physical state and your good looks. But this takes time.

Although you will probably notice a dramatic improvement in how you look and feel and function within the first couple of weeks on biogenics, it may be a few months before any pre-existing subclinical vitamin or mineral deficiencies are cleared up completely and several weeks before the burden of toxicity which you have been carrying has fully cleared. So be patient. The development of the metabolic distortions which caused your original fat-gain has probably taken years. Your body has a quite magnificent ability to heal itself, but this doesn't happen overnight.

Steady Progress vs. a Quick Start
If for the purpose of shedding unwanted fat deposits you were to consult a doctor or health practitioner who uses the biogenic

approach, he or she would – metaphorically speaking – hold your hand throughout the whole process. First you would go through a consultation about how your unwanted fat developed – when and under what circumstances. Then you would probably see him or her maybe once a week or once a fortnight at first, then at longer intervals while he or she gradually taught you the kind of things which are in this book. Most important of all, during your meetings the doctor would constantly monitor your progress and give you the encouragement you needed to make the whole process of fat-shedding as simple and smooth as possible. And, should you hit a rough patch (as we all do from time to time in anything we set out to accomplish), the doctor would be there to reassure you that the processes of nutritional restoration of your body were taking place steadily and slowly, remind you that your fat deposits were melting away, and tell you that before long all would be well.

Unfortunately no book can offer such a service: a book such as this one can neither ask you questions nor adjust itself to your individual needs. All it can hope to do is set down facts and basic principles in a way which, I hope, will enable you to make simple use of them. It can also report on the experiences of others who have been through the biogenic process and wish you the very best should you decide to join them. So bear in mind that this chapter may not apply to you. If this book were a doctor it would tell you to consider all the things in this chapter and then decide for yourself whether or not to do anything about them.

Many people using a book like this one will want to bring about change – particularly the improvement in metabolic processes on which high-level wellbeing and fat-burning depend – as quickly and easily as possible. With this in mind you might consider the possibility of temporarily taking some carefully chosen nutritional supplements which may speed the whole process – especially in the beginning.

While nutritional supplementation is by no means necessary to the success of biogenic fat-loss (indeed most of the natural hygienists would turn over in their graves were one even to suggest such a thing), it can be helpful for people using biogenic techniques without the continual reassurance of a physician. Certain combinations of nutrients can be used to support the processes of detoxification and the restoration of smooth-running metabolic machinery in order that it all happens more quickly. Other nutrients can even be helpful in the reduction of appetite or in the actual process of fat-burning at a cellular level. Whether or not you choose to explore the use of supplemental nutrients is completely up to you. Biogenics will work with or without them. The major drawback they have is that, unlike the diet itself, they tend to be expensive.

I must stress this yet again: *they are in no way essential.* However, because our foods these days are grown on such poor soils, stored for long periods and highly processed, many people develop deficiencies in minerals, trace elements and vitamins which taking specific supplements temporarily can help correct. Biogenics – which depends on foods and exercise alone – is enough in itself. And for many people nutritional supplements would be nothing more than an unwanted and unnecessary expense in what is otherwise quite an inexpensive way of living and eating (sprouts are the best nutritional value for money you will find anywhere). But for others they can help make the whole process of shedding unwanted fat run a little more smoothly. Let's take a look at what nutritional supplementation has to offer.

Anti-Oxidants Aid Spring Cleaning

Anti-oxidants are nutrients – such as vitamins A, C, E, some of the B complex, beta-carotene, zinc, selenium and some of the sulphur-based amino acids – which help protect living systems from the free radical damage that occurs when the body has a high burden of toxicity or is exposed to radiation. Free radicals are formed in your body in a variety of ways. Some are simply by-products of normal metabolic processes. Others come as a result of radiation damage arising, for instance, through exposure to the hazards of low-level nuclear radiation in the environment or electromagnetic emanations from equipment such as video display units of computers or even the ultraviolet rays of the sun. Still others are created through the process of peroxidation whereby the fats or lipids in your body react to form chemical compounds known as peroxides. Whatever their origin, free radicals create toxicity in the system – toxicity which can encourage the laying-down of fat-stores, damage to cells and cell parts, lowering of vitality, cellular pollution, and interference with the healthy metabolic functions which make high-level wellbeing possible.

Anti-oxidant nutrients, as noted, help protect your body from free radical damage. They are master detoxifiers. Each anti-oxidant has a specific action on your body. For instance the water-soluble nutrients such as vitamin C help protect your body's water-soluble molecules, while the oil-based cell membranes in the body get better protection from a fat-soluble anti-oxidant such as vitamin E. But these anti-oxidants – which you take in through the foods you eat and which are also available in higher levels in the form of nutritional supplements – all work in *synergy*. That is, they work together, with the actions of each supporting the actions of many others. And it is the multiple interactions of nutrients – never their single actions – which make them biologically efficient in detoxifying your body and in restoring normal metabolism. Taken three times a day with meals for a few months, a good nutritional formulation of anti-oxidants together with a full range of other vitamins and minerals with which they can work may be of real help to biogenic slimmers. It can hasten the detoxification process of the body. It may also speed the process of restoring nutritional support to the metabolic machinery so that it starts working at peak, for the purpose of fat-burning, much sooner.

A Range of Supplements

Here is a summary of nutritional supplements which may be helpful as adjuncts to your biogenic way of life. Ideally the exact quantity of various nutrients best for you to take in supplementary form is best determined with the help of a doctor well trained in nutrition or a leading-edge nutritionist.

A good anti-oxidant formula including vitamins A, C and E, beta-carotene, biotin, folic acid, calcium pantothenate, vitamins B1, B2, B3, B6 and B12, inositol and PABA (paraaminobenzoic acid) as well as a good balance of essential minerals and trace elements: these may be taken in the form of seaweeds sprinkled on salads or by adding spirulina or green barley, chlorella and green alfalfa or wheatgrass to your soups, or mixing them with water or fruit juice and drinking once a day.

14
Eat and Run

WE'VE SEEN THAT for permanent and lasting fat-loss your metabolic processes need to function at optimal capacity. Thanks to the ability of a diet high in living foods to improve the micro-electrical potentials in cells, to stimulate cell metabolism, to provide a high level of nutrients needed for metabolic pathways to run smoothly, to increase cell oxygenation, and to clear away vitality-sapping wastes from your system, the biogenic system of eating goes a long way in that direction. It can supply both your biochemical and your subtle energy needs for revitalizing living cells. But on its own it is not enough. For, in order to burn fat efficiently, you must also ensure that your cells receive a good supply of oxygen. And that calls for biogenic exercise.

This doesn't mean you have to put on a shiny pink leotard or buy a new jockstrap and head for the gym to wear yourself out. Far from it. But there is truly no point in changing your eating habits unless you also change your living habits by breaking out of the lounge-lizard mould and beginning to go for brisk long walks or swims or jogs at least four times a week. You do not need to become an athlete: you just need regularly and for sustained periods of half an hour to 45 minutes, day after day, to get your heart beating hard and your lungs breathing deeply.

Biogenic exercise is a *gentle* kind of aerobic exercise – a way of exercising which is dependent upon a constant supply of oxygen. It brings more oxygen into your system and it also increases your body's ability to make use of it. The efficiency with which you will discard your unwanted fat-stores depends upon both these things. That's why biogenic fat-loss demands a firm commitment to get out and get moving. But remember the exercise has to be gentle and aerobic to work really well for fat-burning – more about why in the next chapter.

No Help for Lounge Lizards

Oxygen is the vital fuel which burns fat. The fat stored in your cells provides a superb supply of energy, and oxygen is the key for releasing it. The greater your supply of oxygen and the greater your ability to make use of it, the higher your metabolic rate will be and the more success you will have in burning off those unwanted fat-stores.

A major trigger for people to get fat is inactivity. As far back as 1939 an American physician named James Greene surveyed more than 150 obese people about when and under what conditions they had become fat. He discovered that almost 70 per cent of them had grown fat during a period of immobility such as an injury, illness or long convalescence. Only 3 per cent had gained weight simply because they suddenly began to eat more than usual.

What happens to inactive people is that their ability to use oxygen declines and, when it does, their metabolism is lowered. This makes them feel sluggish, encourages the build-up of wastes in their system and, in ways which are as yet not entirely understood scientifically, tends to encourage them to eat all the wrong kinds of things. This is something I have experienced for myself – as have hundreds of other slimmers. You are most inclined to reach for a chocolate bar when you feel both physically and emotionally at your lowest. This experience has a great deal to do with the fact that neither your brain nor the cells in the rest of your body are receiving the oxygen they need to function well and you feel you need energy.

The measurement of how well your body is able to extract oxygen from the environment is expressed in scientific terms as your *VO2max*, or 'maximum oxygen uptake'. In most people this measurement declines steadily after the age of 30 – at a rate of about 1 per cent a year. This decline, and the decline in overall metabolic rate which accompanies it, is a major reason why, as people get older, extra fat-stores tend to creep on. At the same time we lose muscle and bone tissue, our skin wrinkles and thins and we tend to experience a progressive stiffening of the joints. All this takes place not, as scientists once believed, because of time passing but rather because, unlike our primitive ancestors who stayed physically active all through their lives, we lead a largely sedentary existence so that our VO2max declines. And these negative changes occur in exact parallel with the decline in our oxygen-use.

Help for the Hopeless

It is common knowledge that the older you get, particularly if you are a woman, the more difficult it becomes to shed excess fat-stores. I remember a couple of years ago having a conversation with a friend (who is also a highly respected writer on exercise and obesity) and being quite horrified to hear him say to me, 'There is no hope for overweight women over 40 who want to regain their youthful leanness. Their metabolism is simply against them.'

I was shocked – first because I was over 40 myself and I had every intention of shedding my excess fat, and second because I knew in a sense that he was quite right. The combination of fairly high levels of female hormones and a chronically lowered metabolism can be pretty devastating for such women. But he had forgotten two things: first that a biogenic way of eating can transform cellular functioning, enhance vitality and heighten metabolism, and second that when a person of 35 or 40 (or even 70, for that matter) starts getting regular, gentle aerobic exercise – *biogenic* exercise – from taking long walks or runs or steady sustained swims, he or she can, within a matter of a few months, restore VO2max levels to that of someone 20 or more years younger. The body has quite miraculous abilities to restore itself to health given the combination of living foods and a biogenic way of life which includes regular aerobic exercise.

Heightened Metabolism

When you improve your body's use of oxygen through regular exercise your overall metabolic rate increases. This increase can last for many hours after you stop exercising. A study of athletes carried out at the Fatigue Laboratory and the Department of Hygiene at Harvard Medical School showed that 'even fifteen hours after a game or a strenuous practice. . . the metabolic rate is in general distinctly elevated. . . it may be twenty-five per cent above normal'.

The longer you continue to exercise regularly the healthier your metabolism tends to become. This metabolism-stimulating aspect of exercise is an important one to any slimmer. For although on the biogenic diet the tendency for metabolism to drop during a slimming programme is drastically reduced by comparison with the usual low-calorie regime, regular exercise gives you even greater protection from this.

In a weight-reduction programme carried out at the University of California at Davis, researchers found that the fall in metabolic rate which tends to occur with concentrated dieting can be counteracted by putting dieters onto a programme of regular aerobic exercise. For the first two weeks a group of dieters were only put onto a low-calorie regime. As expected, their metabolic rates dropped. They began to experience that sluggish, lacklustre feeling which is so common among dieters and which heralds a slow-down in fat-loss. Then they were put on an exercise programme. Within the next fortnight the metabolic rate of half the dieters had returned to normal (the others were slower to respond). Weight-loss was highest amongst those whose metabolic rates most quickly normalized. In fact one woman actually lost 30 pounds within a month. Weight-loss which is achieved with the help of exercise also protects against those feelings of weakness and heightened nervousness common to slimmers. It replaces them with a sense of strength and relaxation.

How Much? How Long?
To reap the benefits of exercise for weight-loss, to improve your VO2max, heighten your metabolism and keep your spirits high, you need to get the right kind of exercise, you need to take it often enough, and you need to sustain it for long enough periods at each session. A number of studies have been carried out to establish just what the optimum for maximum fat-burning is in each of these respects. Although results differ slightly from one study to another, the general consensus is that you need to exercise aerobically at least four times a week, for at least 40 minutes at each session.

American researchers Leonard Epstein and Rena Wing carried out an analysis of the published data on this subject. They confirmed that the *frequency* of exercise matters greatly. Fatshedders who exercise four or five times a week tend to lose weight up to three times faster than those who exercise only three times a week. Less than three sessions a week were shown to be completely ineffective.

Walking briskly is one of the very best forms of exercise you can get. This doesn't mean a casual stroll but rather a rapid and vigorous walk, regardless of the weather and regardless of whether or not you 'feel like it' at the time. (In fact, when your metabolism *most* needs a boost is when you are likely to feel least like doing it.) Make sure you wear low-heeled shoes and loose comfortable clothing. If you prefer steady swimming or jogging or running or rebounding on a mini-trampoline, by all means go for them instead.

These mini-trampolines which you can use in your own living room while you are watching television, carrying on a conversation or listening to music can be an excellent way of exercising, particularly if you are considerably overweight, since they are fun to use and can be easily adapted to your own particular level of fitness. As you become fitter you simply run on the spot or bounce up and down on them with more force to get a good workout.

How Hard?

The measure of how hard you should work out with whichever form of aerobic activity you choose should come from your heart-rate. This is an easy thing to check by placing two fingers against the artery which surfaces at the wrist just below your thumb and counting your pulse for fifteen seconds, then multiplying by four. This will give you the number of heartbeats per minute, which will tell you how hard your heart is working. If it turns out to be somewhere between 115 and 160 per minute while you are exercising (depending upon your age and condition) then you are exerting yourself to just about the right level. If it is less than that, then you should work harder. If it is more, pull back a little until your heart and lungs get stronger; as this happens you will find you have to exercise harder and harder to give your heart a good workout, but take it easy at first. Your VO2max and your strength will grow rapidly once they begin to alter. Exercising too hard can not only be dangerous if you are not fit, it is also ineffectual for encouraging fat-burning since, under real strain, your muscles switch to an *anaerobic* method of extracting energy which only increases toxicity in the body and interferes with the very oxidation of stored fat which you are trying to achieve. But if you exercise biogenically – slowly, steadily and aerobically – you will be amazed at how much better you look and feel and at how easily even long-term fat deposits can be encouraged to melt away.

Something very important happens when the body is put gently through its paces biogenically over a sustained period of time. After the first half an hour or so of aerobic exercise, instead of your exercise being fuelled by carbohydrate (which has been stored as glycogen in your liver and muscles) your body turns to its fat-stores for fuel. Where in the beginning the cells' energy-burning factories – the mitochondria – could burn carbohydrate fuels, when these become used up the mitochondria use free fatty acids for aerobic burning – provided, of course, there is sufficient oxygen available.

If you start to exercise gently – biogenically – and frequently, by taking long walks or swims or by doing what is known as LSD (long slow distance) running, then your body will learn to switch earlier and earlier from carbohydrate metabolism to fat metabolism. In fact, trained athletes' bodies have learned to metabolize fats almost immediately the exercise starts while sparing their carbohydrate supplies so much that they can go longer and longer at higher speeds with reduced fatigue levels.

The more frequently you exercise and the more devoted you become to ensuring that your body gets the kind of movement it needs and your lungs breathe freely for half an hour to 45 minutes each day, the more easily, quickly and happily you will shed your unwanted body-fat. Besides, although it may be difficult to believe if you are a confirmed lounge lizard, exercise can be *fun*. And even if it is not in the beginning, as you head out of the door on that miserable cold rainy morning feeling as though you can hardly put one foot in front of another, you will end up feeling *great* afterwards. Much of that feeling comes from oxygen – the simple substance you are going to have to teach your body to make better and better use of if you are going to reap all the top benefits of the biogenic diet.

15
Mysteries of Fat-Burning

LET'S LOOK A little more closely at how biogenic exercise works on a biochemical level for lasting fat-loss. Once again, most of it goes back to enzymes.

Fatty acids from fats, amino acids from proteins and glucose from starches are all burnt inside the cells of your muscles to produce energy. This very special cellular burning takes place, as we have seen, in clearly defined steps – thanks to the presence of specific enzymes which make it all happen. This supply of enzymes needed for energy production is dependent upon the cell's genetic material – the DNA – making more enzymes within each cell. This biosynthesis works efficiently only if your cells are well supplied with all the nutrients they need to keep them truly healthy and if they have the proper electrical potentials to encourage it to take place. A biogenic diet comes to the aid of both. So does exercise. For only if you exercise regularly does your DNA get spurred into action. If instead of getting regular aerobic exercise you lead a sedentary life, then, as the tissue proteins and the enzyme proteins (which are the most delicate of all) in your body are being continuously broken down, they cannot be repaired fast enough and your ability to burn calories for energy becomes decreased.

Glucose-Burning vs. Fat-Burning
Glucose is burnt in muscle cells in much the same sort of way as fat, but there are important differences as well. There are a number of metabolic pathways whereby glucose can be broken down by the body's cells, in each case by being first turned into an ester, glucose 6-phosphate. In the metabolic pathway which concerns us, the

glucose 6-phosphate is then converted in muscle cells into fructose 6-phosphate, which is in turn transformed into a chemical called pyruvic acid. Only in the next stage of burning does this pyruvic acid become converted into energy, with water and carbon dioxide as by-products. The enzymes needed to carry out the first stage – breakdown of glucose to give pyruvic acid – need little oxygen to function. However, in the next stage they need a good supply of it; otherwise the pyruvic acid is converted into lactic acid. This is where biogenic exercise comes in.

In biogenic exercise you are continually breathing hard and your heart is beating at up to 80 per cent of its maximum capacity so your muscle cells are well supplied with enough oxygen to carry out both stages in glucose-burning efficiently and simply. But if you exercise too hard – that is, if you allow your heart-rate to go higher than 80 per cent of maximum capacity – then you will be exercising *anaerobically* and depriving your muscle cells of the oxygen they need to carry out the second stage of glucose breakdown (on pages 114–16 we'll look at how to establish just what 80 per cent of your capacity actually is). This is what happens when you end up aching after a workout. The pyruvic acid which your muscle cells have been unable to burn completely into energy has accumulated in your muscles and been changed into lactic acid. This can make them very painful. The fitter you are the more efficiently your cells will grasp the oxygen present in the bloodstream and the less likely you will be to suffer the aches and pains of incomplete glucose metabolism.

Oxygen – A Must for Fat-Burning
When your muscle cells are burning fat, however, the oxygen available to them becomes even more crucial. Fat metabolism, like glucose-burning, takes place in two basic stages but there is a significant difference: in fat-burning all the enzymes involved need a great deal of oxygen all the time. And if you haven't got a sufficient supply of fat-burning enzymes – which fat people, with their sluggish cell metabolism, have not – then unless you change things through biogenic eating and exercise you are likely to get fatter. (Remember that your fat-burning enzymes will increase when you

supply the nutrients for healthy cell functioning and when you stimulate the DNA towards biosynthesis.)

Exercising at 80 per cent capacity or a little less allows you to burn fat while you are in motion as well as stimulating the synthesis of more fat-burning enzymes. But don't decide to push yourself to your limits of energy and endurance on the notion that the harder you exercise the more fat you are likely to burn: you would be making a serious mistake. Exercising at more than 80 per cent of maximum capacity in effect shuts down all fat-burning.

To get your body to produce more fat-burning enzymes and to get these enzymes working hard on your behalf, you need to exercise steadily and slowly, day after day. The more you exercise and the longer you are on the biogenic diet with its ability to improve oxygenation to the cells, then the better your cells will become at grabbing oxygen from the blood and the more and more fat you will burn at higher intensity of movement. But remember, this ability must be built up gradually over a period of time. It doesn't come all at once and it depends on regular biogenic exercise.

Altering Cell Metabolism

Biogenic exercise makes it possible for you to eat more without what you eat turning into fat because it changes your muscle metabolism to that of a fit person. This is very important for permanent fat-loss because it is not only while you are exercising that your muscles burn calories: they also burn 90 per cent of the calories you use up while you are lying around or working at a desk.

The enzymes responsible for burning calories exist only in muscles. So powerful are these enzymes that the muscular movements which go with merely brisk walking can heighten calorie-burning by 50 times over what you burn when you are at rest.

Remember from Chapter 4 that, when you go onto radical low-calorie diets, after the first fortnight (if not before) your cellular metabolism slows down dramatically. This decreases your supply of energy-burning enzymes and therefore your ability to burn calories, so the longer you are on the slimming regime the quicker you are likely to regain your weight afterwards. Low-calorie slimming regimes, unlike exercise and the biogenic diet, are simply incapable of increasing the enzyme supply in your muscles on which calorie-burning depends.

The Magnificent Mitochondria

Most of these enzymes in muscle cells are gathered together in special parts of the cell called the mitochondria – little *organelles* (they look rather like amoebae), sprinkled throughout each cell, which are your cells' powerhouses for energy. It is in the mitochondria that the calorie-burning takes place. Research has shown over and over again that regular aerobic exercise increases not only the number of mitochondria in your cells but also their size as well as the supply of metabolizing enzymes they contain.

In biological terms this is quite simply because people who exercise regularly need more of these energy factories to supply them with fuel to keep going. Such fit people also continue to build more muscle tissue, laying down new cells with yet more energy-burning mitochondria. By contrast, sedentary people who are becoming less and less fit with each passing day are telling their body, in effect, that it really doesn't need these enzymes and so they are not readily replaced when they become depleted. Gradually both the number and size of mitochondria decline as well.

Insulin Sensitivity Needs to Change Too

Other insidious biochemical changes take place in fat people's bodies which make them prone to gaining yet more fat. Some of the most important are the changes which occur to the way they handle insulin and blood sugar. When a fat person eats a meal of refined carbohydrates such as a chocolate bar or a jam sandwich, this causes his or her blood sugar to rise much higher than it does in a fit lean person. The rise in blood sugar is followed by a rise in insulin – the hormone, secreted by the pancreas, whose job it is to control blood-sugar levels. And the rise in insulin also tends to be an unnaturally high one. This is because sedentary fat people have cells which are relatively insensitive to insulin in the bloodstream.

Insulin is important for a number of reasons. Unless enough insulin is present in the circulation, your body's cells cannot take up glucose to be turned into energy even if it is present in good quantity in the blood. They would quite simply starve of this important fuel for life. So how can excess insulin have a deleterious effect?

As people get fat and become unfit, their muscle tissue tends to shrink, cellular metabolic activity falls off and, as part of this process, their cells lose a considerable amount of their ability to respond to insulin in the blood. The presence of insulin normally triggers the opening of certain 'pores' in the cells to allow glucose in, but, since their cells no longer respond normally to the insulin, glucose can enter their muscle cells for energy-burning only very slowly. So blood-glucose levels remain raised longer after each meal they eat. In effect, this glucose left circulating in the blood is on the lookout for some other cells which it can enter . . . and, of course, the kind of cells which are in good supply in fat people are fat cells. The glucose therefore tends to get dumped into these. Once inside them it is converted into glycerol, each molecule of which then attaches itself to three lipid or fat molecules to form a triglyceride – that neutral, stable and extremely hard-to-get-rid-of form of fat which is stored in little droplets throughout the fat cells of your body.

So another major goal of biogenic slimming and biogenic exercise is gradually to tone up muscles, build muscle tissues and increase the sensitivity of muscle cells to insulin. Then, instead of feeling low in vitality because of the difficulty you are having burning glucose for energy, and instead of getting still fatter as glucose is taken into fat cells to be transformed into yet more fat, you will gradually improve your cell metabolism, insulin sensitivity and overall energy levels. As you do so the whole process of shedding fat and then remaining lean – something which in the beginning may have seemed so difficult – gradually becomes easier and easier. In a year or two it will become so much second nature that you will find it difficult to imagine that you ever had a fat problem. But be patient to start with. What has taken you many years to build up in terms of fat deposits and to wind down in terms of slowed metabolism, a poor supply of energy-burning enzymes and too few mitochondria in your cells, will take a little time to change. The important thing with biogenics is, however, that it *will* happen. And you are going to feel wonderful as it does.

16
Your Biogenic Logbook

GETTING INTO EXERCISE is a vital part of the biogenic lifestyle. And it is not difficult to do provided that you set aside some time for it at least four or five times a week and that you don't let your good intentions slip. If you do have any doubts about your health with regard to starting an exercise programme, do seek advice from your doctor before you begin. Whatever exercise you choose to do as your biogenic activity, it must fulfil the following criteria:

- It must be sustained and non-stop.
- It must last at least 40 minutes.
- It must keep your heart beating at about 70 to 80 per cent of its maximum capacity during the whole time you are exercising. (Exercising harder than this will impede fat-burning instead of encouraging it. If you want to get fitter faster, then exercise *longer*, not harder.)
- It needs to be done at least four times a week.

Pick Your Pleasure
The activities you have to choose from are many. But be careful to differentiate between those which are aerobic and those which, because of their stop-start nature, are not. To be biogenic, exercise must be *steady* and *sustained*. Here is a list of various possibilities (by no means exhaustive) to give you some idea of which are aerobic and which anaerobic.

Aerobic Activities	*Anaerobic Activities*
brisk walking	squash
jogging	tennis
LSD (long slow	sprinting
distance) running	
rebounding	golf
cross-country skiing	skiing
cycling	calisthenics
dancing	isometrics
skipping (rope)	badminton
rowing	
swimming	
skating	
circuit-training with weights	

It's Got to be Right for You

If you have the luxury of time to spare then by all means do take up some form of aerobic dance or go to the nearest sports centre and swim laps for 45 minutes each day. But if, like most of us, you have little time, then you are going to have to find other alternatives. One of the best ways to exercise is to take a long brisk walk in comfortable shoes first thing in the morning – even before your biogenic breakfast. You can also walk to work each morning instead of driving or taking the bus or tube. Women can buy themselves a good pair of comfortable training shoes and simply carry their dress shoes with them to put on once they arrive at work. If you have small children and are housebound then perhaps you can get your husband to look after things for 45 minutes while you go out for a walk or a slow steady jog early each morning or after he has returned home in the evening. If your children are small you can put them in a pram or a pushchair and take them on your walk with you; the extra effort of pushing them will do you nothing but good. Or, instead of walking or jogging, you might consider buying a mini-trampoline and using it to bounce or run on the spot in your own living room while you look after your family, listen to music or watch television.

Bounce for Energy

These mini-trampolines (or bouncers) are wonderful inventions. Rebounding on one of these simple contraptions (which can be unobtrusively tucked behind a sofa when not in use) is an excellent form of biogenic exercise for maximum detoxification and metabolic stimulation because of the unique way in which your body, when bouncing, is subjected to the changing force of gravity as it goes up and down. This up-and-down movement, coupled with the concomitant acceleration-deceleration, brings about continual changes in the effective force of gravity exerted on your body. All of your organs, the circulatory and lymphatic systems, and even your individual cells are affected in a way that no other form of exercise accomplishes.

When you are running or skipping on a unit, the G-force at the top of the bounce is effectively non-existent as, for a moment, your body takes on the total weightlessness of an astronaut in space. Then, when you come down again onto the elastic mat, the effective pull of gravity is suddenly increased to two or even three times the usual G-force on earth. This puts the parts of your body under rhythmic pressure.

The kind of cellular stimulation the body receives from this continual gravity/non-gravity exposure stimulates the elimination of wastes from your cells into the interstitial fluid to be carried away through the lymph system and eliminated from the body. Increased oxygen is also brought to the cells to stimulate metabolism. This encourages the steady detoxification of your whole system. The texture of your skin improves, your energy levels rise and, sometimes within only a few days, your body begins to look younger and to feel better.

Stick With It

And, because rebounding is amusing, it is a form of exercise which even lounge lizards usually like. Taking it up one week doesn't usually mean giving it up the next. This fun aspect to rebounding can be important in making sure that you *continue* with the biogenic exercise programme you start. James R. White, a researcher at the University of California at San Diego, designed an interesting study in the long-term effectiveness of weight-loss programmes using exercise. He put some people on rebounders; others rode bicycles; some ran on a treadmill. The control group did nothing but diet. All who exercised regularly and aerobically lost a significant amount of weight and showed a definite increase in the level of their fitness. But in the follow-up study designed to test long-term effectiveness, only 5 per cent of the cyclists and 31 per cent of the runners were still exercising, while a good 58 per cent of the bouncers were still bouncing. This helped keep their metabolic rate high and prevented fat deposits from creeping back on. The explanation the bouncers gave for continuing to exercise was simple. First, rebounding was *easy*. Second, it was fun.

Training Heart-Rate is the Key

Whatever form of aerobic activity you choose, it should raise your heart-rate to 60–75 per cent of maximum. This figure, your 'training heart-rate', is easy to determine. In his excellent book on exercise, *Fit or Fat*, the exercise specialist Covert Bailey describes the way to go about it. However, if you have any doubts at all about your health in regard to your heart, you should always seek a doctor's advice before embarking on a heavy exercise programme.

● Find your Resting Heart-Rate

Three or four times a day, while you are sitting quietly, take your pulse-rate on the artery near the base of your thumb at your wrist for 15 seconds. Multiply this figure by 4 to get your resting pulse-rate. Add up the figures for several readings collected during the day and divide by the number of readings you have made to get your average resting heart-rate. Then write it here:

● Calculate your Maximum Heart-Rate

To do this simply subtract your age from 220. This figure will give you an indication of the fastest your heart can safely beat at your age. (You must *never* exercise at this level!) Write it here:

● Your Training Level

Now you can calculate your training heart-rate – the ideal level at which your heart should beat while you are carrying out your biogenic exercise activity. You *could* simply work out 75 per cent of your maximum heart-rate, but because you are an individual with individual needs you should calculate a more accurate training heart-rate by subtracting your resting heart-rate from your maximum heart-rate, multiplying by 0.65 (i.e., taking 65 per cent of it) and then adding the result back onto your resting heart-rate again. This will give you your training level – the figure you need to remember and to which you must work. Write it here:

● Example
If you are 45 years old and have a resting heart-rate of 70, then the calculations for your training level would go like this:

$$220 - 45 = 175$$
$$(175 - 70) \times 0.65 = 68.25$$
$$68.25 + 70 = 138.25$$

In this case your training level should be below 138 beats a minute for you to get maximum benefits from your exercise. So when you are actually doing your biogenic activity – walking or rebounding or steady swimming or whatever – stop and check your pulse for 15 seconds and multiply by 4 to see that it is at this level. If it is 10 beats per minute (bpm) slower then you need to make more effort. If it is 10 bpm faster, slow down – you are working too hard and not getting your full fat-burning benefits from the activity.

As you continue to exercise over the weeks and months you will find you get fitter and fitter. This means two things. First, your resting pulse itself will tend to drop as your heart becomes stronger and more efficient at delivering blood and oxygen to your cells and tissues (then you will have to update your training level, using the same method to calculate it). And second, you will continually have to work a little harder to keep your pulse-rate at training level. These are both wonderful signs that you are getting the very best out of your biogenic lifestyle . . . but by the time you are recording these changes nobody will have to tell you this – you will feel it yourself.

Log Your Progress
Keep track of your biogenic activity every week to make sure you are spending the time needed to make the most of its ability to stimulate fat-loss and have you living at a very high level of fitness and energy.

The best way to do this is to keep a logbook based on the sample pages shown towards the end of the book on pages 261–6. Each day record the date, the form of exercise you have done, the time you have spent on it and your pulse-rate immediately after you have stopped exercising. Be sure to record your training rate in the little box at the top of each page. Also, make note of the measurements of your waist, hips, left thigh and left upper arm at the end of each month, and also record your weight in the space provided. Your daily logbook, showing a month on each page, will keep you aware of your exercise commitment – and the results at the end of each 30-day period will delight you.

17
Biogenics in Question

TO MOST PEOPLE, embarking on a biogenic lifestyle is a whole new experience. This usually means they have lots of questions they want to ask about it all. Here are the questions I am most frequently asked.

Q: *You say it is not necessary on the biogenic diet to eat flesh foods, and that if they are eaten it should be not more than three times a week. How will I be sure that I am getting enough protein?*
A: It is a common misconception that if you don't eat flesh foods – meat, poultry, fish, seafood and game – or plenty of dairy products such as milk, cheese and eggs, then you won't get enough protein. This is simply untrue. As American biochemist and nutrition expert the late Carl Pfeiffer, author of *Total Nutrition*, says,

> There is a general belief that only meat gives us protein and that vegetables could never be the equal. This is quite erroneous. It is a matter of caloric density: a helping of broccoli has a very high protein value in proportion to the calories consumed. There is also the advantage that the calories are in a high-fibre form.

Meat, like eggs and cheese, is frequently spoken of as being a 'complete' protein. What this means is that it contains all the essential amino acids – those which your body cannot make itself – in a good balance so that once the meat's protein is broken down into these amino acids it provides your system with the raw materials needed to repair its own proteins, make new enzymes and hormones, and build muscle tissue. For many years most nutritionists believed that it was necessary to take in all of the essential amino acids at each meal in order to make proper use of them. Now we know that this is not so. Eating as you do on the biogenic diet you can take in all of the essential amino acids at one meal – for instance in the combination of a biogenic salad served with a seed cheese or starch soup – or you can take in some essential amino acids at one meal and others at another meal. Your body will still be able with ease to make use of these free aminos to build proteins. This is because all these aminos become part of what is known as your 'amino-acid pool', which is, in effect, your own readily available bank of free aminos on which your body can draw when it needs to build proteins in the body. But you do not have to take them all at one meal. You will get the same protein-building abilities if the foods are consumed within a 24-hour period.

The question of exactly how much protein you need for high-level health is one which can provoke heated argument. Early recommendations hovered at between 120g and 160g a day, although as long ago as the turn of the century scientists had shown that you could actually live more healthily on half that and other studies have since indicated that good health is possible on as little as 20g a day. Dr. Myron Winick of the Institute of Human Nutrition at Columbia University School of Medicine has studied this question thoroughly and says that for maximum protection against premature ageing and degeneration the 'recommended daily intake for healthy adult men and women of almost any age is 56 grams and 46 grams respectively'. On the biogenic diet you will certainly get that – although, because the diet is rich in a variety of vegetable foods, you are likely to need even less protein. For it is not just the *quantity* that matters but *quality*. And the quality of protein in such a mixed vegetable diet, with some 70 per cent of your foods eaten raw to supply all eight essential amino acids in easily assimilable form, is very high indeed.

In fact, the biogenic diet is *moderate* in protein. This is for a very good reason: too much protein can be dangerous. A diet which supplies more protein than your body needs can cause severe deficiencies of many essential vitamins, including vitamins B6 (pyridoxine) and niacin. Excess protein actually leaches important minerals such as calcium, iron, zinc, phosphorus and magnesium from your body. And, when your body metabolizes protein, complex by-products are formed, some of which (such as ammonia) can be highly toxic to the system, encouraging free radical damage and stressing your body. This kind of toxicity especially needs to be avoided in order to encourage fat-shedding. Many animal studies have now shown conclusively that, while a high-protein diet brings about early rapid growth, it also results in early and rapid ageing and degeneration. You want to avoid it.

Q: *How fast will I lose weight on the biogenic programme?*
A: That depends upon the idiosyncrasies of your own metabolism, on how long you exercise and on how rapidly your body detoxifies itself. In the beginning you are likely to lose weight very quickly, but this initial weight-loss will be not fat but water as your system begins to clear of toxicity. (Wastes in the tissues encourage the body to retain water in order to dilute them and render them less dangerous.) It is best to aim for no more than two pounds a week. This way you give your body time to change gradually: you neither risk your system being flooded with toxicity (which can make you want to eat foods in combinations you should avoid) and nor do you trigger the setpoint mechanism to try to replace fat which has already been shed.

In fact, you may not have any choice in the matter: many people following a biogenic lifestyle lose weight *much* faster. If this is the case with you, then, to slow things down a bit, you might avoid applefasting even one day a week and make sure that at least 30 per cent of the foods you eat are cooked (another way of helping slow down fat-loss). Provided you get your full quota of biogenic exercise, however, you should not have to worry too much if you are shedding fat at a rate faster than two pounds a week. Taking lots of exercise goes a long way towards adjusting the setpoint and eliminates toxicity with great efficiency.

Q: *The biogenic diet contains a lot of raw foods and I understand that raw foods are more difficult to digest. Will they give me problems such as flatulence or loose bowels?*
A: This is a common misconception. In fact raw foods, provided they are well chewed, are *less* difficult to digest than their

counterparts: this is why they form the basis of traditional dietary treatments in natural medicine. Remember, these uncooked foods are rich in enzymes which render them almost self-digesting. They take a great deal of strain off your digestive enzymes. As far as causing flatulence is concerned, this does occasionally happen in the beginning but only to a few people. And it shouldn't happen at all if you are combining your foods properly. If it does you might suspect dysbiosis – undesirable flora in the intestines, such as *Candida albicans*, a condition which may need treatment (see page 63).

When it comes to loose bowels, the answer is twofold. Firstly, in the beginning you may find – particularly if you choose to do an applefast – that you have extremely loose bowels. This is an indication that your body is very rapidly clearing away its wastes. The condition should stop within a day or two. Secondly, later on you will discover that you are having a considerable number of bowel movements – maybe two or three a day when before you had only one. This is a good sign: it means that your digestion and elimination processes are working properly. Researchers find the same thing among primitive peoples living on a healthy diet of natural unrefined foods and among children raised on the same sort of diet.

Q: *How expensive is a biogenic way of eating?*

A: Like an ordinary diet it can be either expensive or inexpensive depending on how much you have to spend and what kind of foods you choose to buy. Obviously if you are going to munch mangoes for breakfast and use exotic vegetables for your salads, soups and other dishes, it can be pricey. On the other hand, using the fruits and vegetables which are readily available in season, it can be very inexpensive indeed. The best of the biogenic foods – sprouted seeds and grains – are among the most inexpensive foods you can buy anywhere as well as being of the highest nutritional value. Living on the biogenic diet can be *considerably* cheaper than if you're living on the diet of processed convenience foods which the majority of people eat.

Q: *Do I have to eat three meals a day? In other words, do I have to eat every meal even if I'm not hungry?*

A: No, you don't. But you need to make sure that the foods in each meal you *do* eat are properly combined and that you have left plenty of time (four to five hours) after a protein or starch meal for it to be completely digested before you eat anything else. Many people find, after a week or two on the biogenic diet, that their appetite decreases dramatically. If this is the case by all means skip a meal or opt for a piece of fruit or a yogurt drink in its place.

PART TWO

THE PRACTICE

18
Ready Steady Go

NOW THAT YOU'VE met the principles, it's time to immerse yourself in the practice of biogenics. This is where all the fun begins. For, unlike the usual low-calorie regime with its minute portions of processed foods, the biogenic diet offers you as much as you want to eat from nature's cornucopia of delights. The beauty and the texture of fresh foods prepared in simple yet attractive ways is, for me, one of the great pleasures of life. When I first began exploring biogenics for myself I was amazed to discover three things. Firstly, these foods which were so good for me were also more delicious than any I had eaten before. Secondly, they were simple to prepare. Finally, this biogenic way of eating offered such an extraordinary variety of taste, aroma, colour and texture that I was never bored.

During my first month of practising biogenics I shed a stone of excess fat. My cheekbones, which for several years had been largely hidden beneath a little too much cushion on my face, suddenly emerged and my face as a whole took on a new and younger shape. My clothes began to hang on me. When I went out for a run I noticed that my movements had become more fluid and my step lighter. And all I had been doing was following the biogenic guidelines for conscientious food combining, chewing my foods until every morsel of flavour had been gleaned from them, and eating absolutely as much as I wanted.

Metamorphosis
Biogenics is far more than just a programme for weight-loss: it is a lifestyle for high-level wellbeing – a way of living that will help

prevent premature ageing, illness and fatigue. And it is not something which you follow for a period of weeks until you have shed your excess fat, then return to the same old eating habits which caused you the fat problem in the first place. Think of the biogenic experience which you will be having in the next few weeks as a transition between the way you *were* living and a better, more energetic and satisfying lifestyle of the future – a lifestyle which will protect you permanently from ever having to deal with a fat problem again. During the next few weeks you will be going through a kind of metamorphosis which will help balance your body's biochemical functioning and put you in harmony with your natural body-cycles. Once this metamorphosis has started, the process of detoxification will continue uninterrupted. And, so long as you continue to make the biogenic principles the guidelines by which you live, fat-loss will take place automatically – as a natural consequence of the whole process – until your body happily readjusts itself to its most comfortable and natural weight. One of the great blessings of this metamorphosis is that the further along you are in the change process, the more energy and initiative you will find you have to continue. It is rather like getting yourself into the opposite of a vicious circle: each positive thing that you do reinforces yet further positive change.

Flesh Foods By Choice

In chapters 21–9 of this book you will find recipes for soups, salads, dips and dressings, vegetable dishes and all the other basic dishes which fit easily into the biogenic way of living. You will not, however, find recipes for fish, poultry, game, seafood and eggs for two reasons. First most people already know how to prepare these foods. Second, although they are foods which you should by all means eat and enjoy if you want to, they are in no way *essential* to the transformation which will be taking place within the next few weeks. Indeed, eating too many flesh foods or eating them too often may interfere with the detoxification process. However, if you enjoy them by all means eat them – but make sure that they are prepared simply, without the addition of starch-based sauces, and make sure you eat only one flesh food at a meal. The best way to prepare flesh foods is, as I say, simply – by grilling, baking or poaching.

Eggs can be made into delicious omelettes or hard-boiled and then grated and sprinkled on your salads. At our home in Pembrokeshire we used to keep our own chickens who provided us with far more superb free-range eggs than we could ever eat. Now I buy free-range organic eggs.

You can create your own delicious dishes by combining eggs or flesh foods with light crisp salads and serving them hot or cold. But remember that you don't want to eat flesh foods more than three or four times a week. They are very concentrated proteins and also low-water foods. Don't forget that for effective detoxification and efficient fat-loss you need to make sure that 70 per cent of what you eat comes from the high-water foods such as fresh raw fruits and vegetables and biogenic sprouts.

The Biogenic Kitchen

Most of the things you need in order to prepare delicious recipes for your new biogenic lifestyle are things which you probably already have in your kitchen. The one machine I consider essential is a food processor. You can get by without a blender as the food processor can do many of the same things but, if you happen to have one, it too can be useful. When buying either, it is most important that you buy good, strong machines which will stand up to heavy demands; if you have a fairly large family it is sometimes worth investing in the catering or industrial models as they are more sturdily made and have a greater capacity.

If you can afford it you might consider buying a juice extractor – this can be a wonderful tool for producing delicious and vibrant fruit and vegetable cocktails. But gadgets like the juice extractor are really the icing on the cake and in no way necessary to preparing your foods. Here are a few guidelines if you decide to buy any of these machines.

Food Processors

A good food processor is a real blessing to a biogenic lifestyle. These machines have many varied and remarkable attachments including, usually, a blade, several graters of different sizes, slicers and shredders. The blade attachment is great for grinding nuts, seeds and wheat and other sprouts, homogenizing vegetables for soups and loaves, and making dressings and dips. In fact, many of these can also be done in the blender, but if they are gooey they tend to get stuck around the blade and you can spend five minutes trying to scrape out your dessert with very little to show for it. The blade of the food processor, by contrast, is removable and easy to scrape, so you lose very little.

The other food-processor attachments are terrific for making salads. You can prepare a splendid biogenic salad in about five minutes with the help of these friends. Experiment with grating, finely slicing and shredding all kinds of vegetables because, believe it or not, vegetables actually taste different depending on how they are cut up!

Blenders

Blenders do not differ greatly except in power. But look for one which is at least 400 watts (any less will be unable to cope). Some can be bought with attachments for grating, chopping, kneading, etc., which are very useful. Glass bowls are preferable to plastic ones as the plastic tends to stain and look tatty very quickly (and those stains are more than likely to be harbouring bacteria). A removable blade (the base unscrews) can make cleaning easier. I like the hand-held blenders too. They are not so strong but great for purées or soups or blending juice with green substances like spirulina to make green drinks.

Juicers

The most important considerations when selecting a juicer are power, capacity, and ease of cleaning – some have a removable strip of plastic gauze in the pulp basket which is helpful in cleaning. In general, the fewer fiddly parts to wash up the better. As with blenders, some juicers have additional attachments.

Juicers vary greatly and can be a pleasure or a bind to use. There are basically two types: hydraulic-press juicers and centrifugal juicers. Some hydraulic presses are hand-operated and therefore less convenient than the electric juicers, but a few doctors who work with raw juices prefer them because they believe they reduce the amount of oxidation that takes place when the juice is exposed to the air. We have a centrifugal juicer ourselves. Of the centrifugal juicers there are two types: the separators, which operate continuously, and the batch operators, which have to be cleaned out after about two pounds of material have been juiced.

Separators are the more convenient of the two because they do not fill up with the vegetable/fruit pulp, but expel it. However, they tend not to extract juice as efficiently as the batch operators, so that you might find you want to re-juice the expelled pulp.

Some batch juicers are better than others. It is best to look for a large-capacity one which requires only infrequent emptying. It can be extremely tiresome to contend with a machine that insists on being cleaned out after juicing only half a glass when you are juicing for six people!

Citrus-Fruit Juicer

The juicer consists of a rotating central form onto which you press the halved fruit. You use it to make orange, grapefruit or lemon juice very quickly and easily. Of course, these fruits can also be juiced in a centrifuge juicer, but they need to be peeled first, which is time-consuming.

Lettuce Spin-Drier

The lettuce spin-drier is a great invention. There are several types, but my favourite consists of a basket which holds the lettuce (or other greens) and fits into a container with holes in the bottom and a lid with a cord attached. The lid has a hole in the top. You put the device into your sink and run water slowly into the hole in the lid while pulling the cord repeatedly. This spins the basket and expels the water, in theory cleaning and drying the greens. In practice, however, the leaves often need to be rinsed clean before being put into the basket; but by spinning them dry you get beautifully crisp fresh greens very quickly.

Hand-Powered Alternatives

The following are helpful if you don't have a food processor and a lot of other electrical equipment. However, you may find that using these hand-powered alternatives you are a little limited in the variety of recipes you are able to prepare.

- Food processors: there are several hand-operated types which perform either chopping functions or grating/slicing, etc.; some are rather cheaply made, so look out for a sturdy one.
- Hand meat/grain grinder or coffee grinder: for mincing grains and grinding seeds and nuts.
- Pestle and mortar: for grinding herbs, spices, etc.
- Hand grater: the box kind with several different facets is best.
- Citrus reamer: the well-known 'lemon squeezer'.
- Salad basket: the kind made of wire which you take outside and swing around your head.

In a biogenic lifestyle, the things that matter most are of course the foods themselves. And there are so many different ways of preparing them that you can probably turn the lack of a food processor or other equipment to your advantage if you let it push you towards discovering even more creative ways of serving the splendid natural foods which you will be eating.

Look Ahead

The following chapters contain scores of recipes for you to sample. I hope that they will serve as inspiration to you to create your own; if you do I would love to hear about them. The recipes are simple and portions in them are loosely defined: most will serve about four people. I encourage you to cut them in half, alter them in any way you fancy to include your own favourite ingredients, and even enlarge them if you wish when you feel particularly hungry and want to eat more. But remember that you must always chew your foods *completely* so that you get every morsel of pleasure you can out of them. Remember, too, that you must stop eating immediately when your appetite signals to you that you've had enough. DO NOT OVEREAT.

Look on the next few weeks as a period of transition, take a deep breath and make the leap into biogenics.

Here we go.

19
The Daily Dozen

HERE ARE 12 basic guidelines for biogenic living. They are the principles to which you will refer frequently in the beginning. Before long, however, they will become second nature. Included in this section as well is a quick reference chart on food combining which shows what goes with what.

1. Never Mix Concentrated Proteins with Concentrated Starches

The old days of meat-and-potatoes or fish-and-chips are something you want to leave behind. Concentrated protein foods such as nuts, seeds, dairy products, eggs and flesh foods need an acid medium for efficient digestion, while concentrated starches such as beans and grains, potatoes, breads, cereals, yams and pumpkins need an alkaline one. When these foods are mixed it delays digestion, tends to produce toxicity in the system and is responsible both for increasing appetite and digestive upsets. What you can get away with is the occasional garnish of protein foods or fruit foods – such as sesame seeds or raisins – in a dish to which you would never add them in greater quantity.

2. Eat Fruit on Its Own

Fruit passes through your digestive system very rapidly and requires little action by digestive enzymes in order to break it down for bodily use. If fruit is eaten at a meal with other foods its digestion and assimilation are slowed drastically and you can get fermentation in the gut. This results in indigestion, wind and discomfort; some people find that fruits eaten this way can turn into alcohol in their stomach, and this affects mind and mood. If you want to eat fruit with other food use it as a starter and be sure to leave 20–30 minutes for its digestion before beginning your second course. However, acid fruits can be eaten with nuts to create a meal for lunch or supper. And both the acid and sub-acid fruits can be eaten with cottage cheese. Sweet fruits such as bananas, raisins, dates, figs and prunes should never be put into a salad which has a concentrated protein in it. The one fruit which is rather unique in that it will combine quite well with raw vegetables in salads is apple.

3. Eat Only Fruit for Breakfast

Breakfast must be an entirely fruit meal. You may eat as much as you like (provided you listen carefully to the dictates of your appetite and you masticate even the softest of fruits until the last bit of sweetness is extracted from them). Your liver – the body's most important organ for detoxification – is most active between midnight and midday. Eating fruit (which is virtually self-digesting), unlike taking in starch or protein foods, allows this detoxification process to continue unimpeded. All other foods interfere with it. You may have more fruit mid-morning if you are hungry; this will only aid in the whole process. But make sure you leave a gap of at least 20 to 30 minutes (45 minutes for a banana) before you begin your midday meal. You must leave 4–5 hours after a main starch or protein meal before eating fruit again and do not drink fruit juice between meals (except as a starter leaving plenty of time before the rest of your meal, or as a mid-morning snack if you wish).

4. Go for a Biogenic Salad Once a Day

The biogenic salad based on home-grown or store-bought sprouted seeds and grains is the mainstay of the biogenic lifestyle. (Remember, biogenic foods should form 20 to 40 per cent of what you eat each day.) While it is by no means absolutely essential that you base one of your meals each day on a biogenic salad, this is the best possible way to get optimal support for rebuilding cells and tissues, rebalancing biochemical processes, and restoring normal metabolism. Sometimes of course this is not possible – for example, when you are having to eat in restaurants all the time – but then you can replace the biogenic salad with a big bioactive dish (bioactive foods should make up between 35 and 50 per cent of what you eat each day) full of fresh vegetables and served with a side-dish of grains, a soup or a protein food or simply with a couple of slices of wholegrain bread. But the more often you are able to make a biogenic salad the focus of the meal the sooner you will reap the rewards of your new biogenic lifestyle.

5. Make Your Foods the Very Best You Can Get

This doesn't mean spending lots of money on them: it means being fussy when you go to the greengrocer and always choosing foods which are fresh, as much as possible whole (such as wholegrains), and eaten as close as possible to their natural state.

6. Steer Clear of *Biocidic* Foods

The biocidic foods which have been excessively processed to alter their natural state are depleted of nutrients and tend to contain potentially harmful additives such as artificial colourings and flavourings. They include foods such as white breads, sugars, most meats, sweets, coffee and most of the ready-in-a-minute convenience foods that fill the shelves of our supermarkets. These are the most polluting of all foods. They have no place on the biogenic table.

7. Make Biostatics Your Side-Dishes

Biostatic foods are energy foods. They include wholegrains and cooked vegetables, legumes and dairy products, fresh fish, poultry and game. These foods are both delicious and satisfying. They are good sources of sustained energy (particularly the grains) and useful as a provider of proteins for the body's amino-acid pool. They also make a beautiful contrast to the lighter, finer taste and feel of the biogenics and the bioactives. Use them with pleasure but also in moderation. The best way to do this is to serve them as side-dishes at your meals. This is a brand new and very healthy twist to the traditional practice of making meat and cooked vegetables the focus of a meal which is then eaten with a side-salad. In the biogenic system these cooked foods become the side-dishes to complement biogenic and bioactive main recipes.

Biostatic foods should make up about 25 per cent of what you eat each day.

8. Swim with the Water Margin
Your body is 70 per cent water. For it to detoxify itself and to encourage the restoration of normal functioning on a cellular level as well as in the system as a whole, 70 per cent of what you eat each day needs to be chosen from the high-water foods: fresh fruits, sprouts, and vegetables eaten raw. This is probable the easiest guideline of all to keep to, for when you are having only fruit for breakfast and making one meal a day a biogenic or bioactive main-course salad it just about takes care of itself. But there may be days when you find you have eaten more biostatic foods than you should because of being invited out or having to eat in restaurants. Then it is a good idea to make the next day an all-raw day where you have fruit for breakfast as usual, a biogenic dish for lunch, and then another fruit dish or a bioactive dish for dinner.

9. Do Not Eat Between Meals
(Except, that is, between breakfast and lunch if you are really hungry.) Your digestive system absolutely must have time to complete the digestion of a meal before you put anything else into it. This means four or five hours need to elapse between lunch and dinner. Otherwise digestion is not complete and increased toxicity can ensue. Do drink spring water or herb teas between meals if you like. And if a meal is delayed beyond four or five hours after your last meal you can have a piece of fruit or two to tide you over. Otherwise stick carefully to your mealtimes.

10. Choose Your Condiments
Begin reading labels on what you buy and make sure that any commercial salad dressings, condiments and seasonings that you buy contain no chemical additives, sugar or preservatives. They will only increase the toxicity in your body. Use raw honey for sweetening and then only occasionally and in small quantities.

11. Be Creative
Don't forget that the suggested biogenic menus which follow are

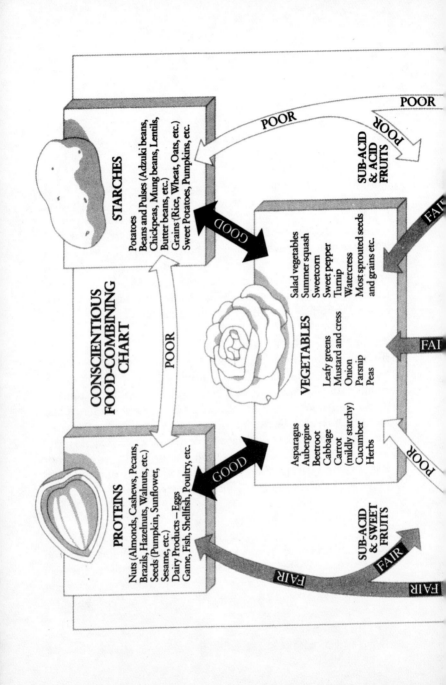

CONSCIENTIOUS FOOD-COMBINING CHART

STARCHES

Potatoes
Beans and Pulses (Adzuki beans,
Chickpeas, Mung beans, Lentils,
Butter beans, etc.)
Grains (Rice, Wheat, Oats, etc.)
Sweet Potatoes, Pumpkins, etc.

PROTEINS

Nuts (Almonds, Cashews, Pecans,
Brazils, Hazelnuts, Walnuts, etc.)
Seeds (Pumpkin, Sunflower,
Sesame, etc.)
Dairy Products – Eggs
Game, Fish, Shellfish, Poultry, etc.

VEGETABLES

Salad vegetables
Summer squash
Sweetcorn
Sweet pepper
Turnip
Watercress
Most sprouted seeds
and grains etc.

Leafy greens
Mustard and cress
Onion
Parsnip
Peas

Asparagus
Aubergine
Beetroot
Cabbage
Carrot
(mildly starchy)
Cucumber
Herbs

SUB-ACID & ACID FRUITS

SUB-ACID & SWEET FRUITS

GOOD

GOOD

GOOD

POOR

POOR

POOR

POOR

FAIR

FAIR

FAIR

FAIR

POOR

SWEET FRUITS

Banana
Dates
Dried figs
Persimmon
Raisins and other dried fruits
Etc.

SUB-ACID FRUITS

Apple   Nectarine
Apricot   Papaya
Blackcurrants Peach
Fresh figs   Pear
Grapes   Sweet Cherries
Kiwi fruit   Etc.
Mango

ACID FRUITS

Blackberries   Pomegranate
Grapefruit   Raspberries
Lemon   Satsuma
Lime   Strawberries
Orange   Tangerine Etc.
Pineapple
Plum

FAIR (between Sub-Acid and Sweet Fruits)

GOOD (between Acid and Sub-Acid Fruits)

FAIR (between Acid/Sub-Acid and Sweet Fruits)

NEUTRAL FOODS

(they go well with anything)

Avocado   Olives   Seed oils

RECOMMENDATION

All juices can be mixed because they are liquid and can be absorbed by the body within half an hour

COMBINATIONS

Fruit & Starch
Protein & Starch

Leafy greens & Acid fruits
Leafy greens &
Protein & Acid fruits

Avocado & Acid or
Sub-acid fruits
Avocado & Leafy vegetables
Protein & Leafy greens
Starch & Vegetables
Oils & Leafy greens
Oils & Acid or Sub-acid fruits

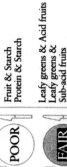

POOR

FAIR

GOOD

MELONS

(eat on their own or leave alone)

Cantaloupe Honeydew Watermelon
Crenshaw   Ogen   Etc.

RECOMMENDATION

Make meals of one or two combinations, especially of one protein or one starch with one or two vegetables

merely guidelines. Play about with them and make them your own. Figure out ways of getting your favourite foods into your meals. You might be surprised to find just how many of the recipes in the section which follow will appeal to others in your family as well. If you make a biogenic salad for yourself make a little side-salad just like it to go with the chop you may be cooking for your husband. Many a family member has been gently drawn into a healthier way of eating and living by taste alone. Never preach. Have fun with it all. If you do it may well eventually turn out to be fun for the rest of your family as well.

12. Make Time for Exercise

Be good to yourself and make sure that, no matter what kind of mountains you may have to move to do it, you set aside a space in your life of at least 30 minutes in a day, four times a week, for biogenic exercise. This is an absolute must. In due course it will become an absolute joy as well. But it means making the effort *now* to make it possible.

Take a close look at the conscientious food-combining chart on the previous two pages. Use it like a map to steer you through the new territory of your biogenic lifestyle.

20
Shopping Spree

NOW IT IS time, with biogenic principles in mind, to think about stocking your larder. Many of the foods you will be using on the biogenic diet you probably already have. Others can be found in supermarkets, healthfood stores and wholefood emporiums. And of course most of the fresh foods are readily available at your supermarket or local greengrocer. The sprouts you will use for your biogenic salads can be bought in some supermarkets and in healthfood stores. But they are so much more delicious if you grow them yourself (see pages 186–7).

You'll find that the list of fresh wholesome food from which you can choose for the biogenic diet is very large indeed. It contains over 150 quite common foods and, of course, there are many more if you take into consideration the herbs, the wild salad foods, and the more exotic fruits and nuts which you can get if you want to take the trouble to look for them.

Let's take a closer look at some of the different types of food which are available and the specific foods that you may want to choose from to create a biogenic way of eating for lasting fat-loss.

Fresh Fruits
The 'great eliminators', fresh fruits are high in vitamins, minerals and enzymes, all of which help detoxify your system at a rapid rate. The gentle acidity of most fruits can dissolve waste substances in the tissues and help carry them away. Fruit also helps stimulate metabolism. Make at least one meal a day an entirely fruit meal. And for maximum weight-loss it is a good idea to spend at least one day a week detoxifying your body on a single fruit. Probably the best

fruit (in a temperate climate like Britain) to use is the apple (see details of the applefast on pages 88–93). Fruits to choose from include:

apple	mango
apricot	mulberries
banana	nectarine
berries	ogen melon
blackberries	orange
blackcurrants	pawpaw (papaya)
blueberries	peach
cantaloupe melon	pear
cherries	Persian melon
cranberries	persimmon
Crenshaw melon	pineapple
fresh figs	plum
gooseberries	pomegranate
grapefruit	prunes
grapes	raspberries
honeydew melon	redcurrants
kiwi fruit	satsuma
kumquat	strawberries
lemon	tamarind
lime	tangerine
lychees	watermelon

Vegetable Fruits

Bioactive foods such as avocados, tomatoes, peppers and cucumber are actually classified botanically as fruits. However, they are most frequently used as vegetables. In fact they do combine well with other fruits. You can put avocado together with mango, for instance, or cucumber together with oranges very successfully. These vegetable fruits also combine well with neutral vegetables and with the starchy carbohydrates such as rice, other grains, and potatoes.

The vegetable fruits are best eaten raw. Except for the avocado they tend, like most fruits, to pass through the stomach very quickly. The vegetable fruits are:

avocado

peppers (red, green, yellow)

cucumber

tomatoes

Fresh Raw Vegetables

These foods contain important organic minerals and vitamins. They too help eliminate stored toxicity in the system. Each day you can eat as much raw salad as you like. You can use these foods to supply the necessary minerals such as calcium and iron as well.

Generally speaking most vegetables mix well, both with concentrated proteins and with concentrated starches. Those which are stored (rather than eaten fresh), however, are very high in starch and should be used only for starch meals. Recommended fresh raw vegetables include:

alfalfa sprouts	lamb's lettuce
artichokes	leeks
asparagus	lettuce (all kinds)
bean sprouts	marrow
beetroot	mung bean sprouts
beet greens	mustard greens
Brussels sprouts	mushrooms
cabbage	onion
carrots	okra
cauliflower	parsley
celery	parsnip
Chinese leaves	peas (green or mange-tout)
chives	potatoes
collards	pumpkin
corn-on-the-cob	radish sprouts
dandelion leaves	radishes
dill	salsify
endive	scallions (shallots)
fenugreek sprouts	spinach
garlic	spring onions
green beans	sweet potato
Jerusalem artichoke	Swiss chard
kale	turnip
kohlrabi	turnip greens

yam   watercress
yellow beans

Sea Vegetables

If you have never used the sea vegetables for cooking, this is an ideal time to begin. Not only are they delicious – imparting a wonderful, spicy flavour to soups and salads – they are also the richest source of organic mineral salts in nature, particularly of iodine. Iodine is the mineral which is necessary in order for the thyroid gland to work efficiently. As your thyroid gland is largely responsible for the body's metabolic rate, iodine is very important for slimmers.

I like to use powdered kelp as a seasoning. You will find it in some of the recipes. In fact, I use it in many more – to add both flavour and minerals to salad dressings, salads, soups and so forth. I am also very fond of nori seaweed, which comes in long thin sheets. It is a delicious snack food which you can eat along with a salad or at the beginning of the meal: it has a beautiful, crisp flavour. I like to toast it very, very quickly by putting it under a grill for no more than 10 or 15 seconds. It is also delicious raw.

Get to know some of the sea vegetables and begin to make use of them. Your nails and hair will be strengthened by the full range of minerals and trace elements such as selenium, calcium, iodine, boron, potassium, magnesium, iron and others which are not always found in great quantities in our ordinary garden vegetables. So will the rest of your body.

You can use nori seaweed to wrap around everything from a sprout salad to cooked grains in order to make little pieces of vegetarian *sushi*. It's often a good idea to soak some of the other sea vegetables such as dulse, arrame and hiziki for a few minutes in enough tepid water to cover. This softens them so that they can be easily chopped to be put into salads or added to soups. Sea vegetables are available in healthfood stores and in oriental food shops. Recommended ones are:

arrame   dulse
hiziki   kelp
kombu   laver bread
nori   wakami

Foods to Sprout

The sprouted seeds, grains and legumes are truly life-generating and are the very basis of the biogenic diet. These foods contain life- and health-enhancing energies which appear to potentialize and mobilize dormant life forces in the animal organism eating them. At least one meal a day should consist of a large biogenic dish. This can be a large soup or a salad containing the sprouted seeds and the grains or both. See the sprouting chart on pages 186–7. Recommended seeds/grains/pulses/nuts for sprouting include:

adzuki (aduki)	mung
alfalfa	mustardseed
almond	oats
barley	radish
buckwheat	rye
chickpea	sesame
cress	sunflower
curly cress	triticale
lentil	watercress
maize	wheat
millet	

Nuts and Seeds

These biogenic foods are very concentrated sources of body-building protein and are also rich in natural oils. They should be eaten regularly as part of the biogenic diet but never in great quantities. They are more difficult to digest than fresh fruits and vegetables and are often best used chopped very finely and sprinkled onto salads or mixed with a little spring or filtered water in order to make a nut sauce which can then be served over salads, soups and even some fruits (see food-combining chart on pages 136–7). When you're eating nuts or seeds at any meal do not eat any other concentrated foods. Excellent ways of rendering them more digestible are to ferment them or to soak them overnight. Try these:

almonds	pine kernels
brazils	poppy seeds
caraway seeds	pumpkin seeds
cashews	sesame seeds
coconuts	sunflower seeds
hazelnuts	marrow seeds
pecans	walnuts

You will notice that peanuts (groundnuts) are not listed here. This is because they are in fact legumes and not nuts at all. They are an excellent source of vitamin B3 and biotin but are also very acid-forming. They should be treated as a concentrated protein and eaten only in small quantities, always raw, never roasted and never heavily salted.

Grains

Grains were the first food which man cultivated, and they have formed a major staple ever since. They are not strongly eliminative but they are well-balanced foods that contain the nutrients needed for good health – particularly the B-complex vitamins. Wholegrains are also an excellent source of fibre and of sustainable energy. They are important foods for athletes and for very active people.

On the biogenic diet you can include your 'quota' of grains by preparing side-dishes such as millet, brown rice, buckwheat (a seed rather than a grain but often classified together with the grains) or wholemeal pasta to go with your vegetables and salads. Or you can eat a slice or two of any good wholegrain bread with your neutral or starch meal. Most slimmers find that they are better off eating rye or pumpernickel breads – the European darker, heavier, natural breads – than the usual wholewheat. This is because wheat contains a high percentage of gluten which in many people tends to clog the intestines. Despite its quite high bran content, wholemeal bread can cause intestinal discomfort that leads to excess appetite and also, surprisingly, to constipation in some people. There are also some excellent grain breads and crackers on the market which you can buy.

The grains themselves make wonderful additions to starch soups or cooked on their own as a side-dish.

Recommended breads and biscuits include:

wholegrain pitta bread	rye crisp
pumpernickel bread	100 per cent rye
home-made bran muffins	Scottish oatcakes
wholecorn tortillas	wholegrain chapatis

Recommended grains and grain products include:

barley	kasha
bulgar wheat	millet
corn meal	pasta (wholegrain)
couscous	rice (brown)

Legumes

The legumes/pulses are unusual foods in nature in that many of them are both concentrated starches and proteins. As such (with the exception of lentils) they can be quite difficult for many slimmers to digest. Therefore on the biogenic slimming diet few legumes are used – except, of course, in sprouted form. The one which is commonly used unsprouted is the lentil – red, brown, green or black.

Legumes often contain a trypsin inhibitor, a substance which blocks the action of some of the enzymes which break down protein in your body. Because of this, legumes should never be eaten raw, because then a proportion of the valuable amino acids they contain cannot be used. Trypsin inhibitors are destroyed when the legumes are cooked, and sprouting neutralizes the trypsin inhibitors as well. (The sprouting of lentils and other legumes and grains also destroys other harmful substances such as phytic acid [see page 86].)

Tofu – soybean curd – is a very high-protein food which is low in fat and much favoured in the Orient. It can make an interesting addition to a salad dressing or as the basis of a protein salad.

Dairy Products

Ideally any dairy products that you eat on the biogenic diet should be unpasteurized and low in fat. This is becoming extremely difficult in Britain. However, there are some excellent unpasteurized goats' milks available from which you can make goats' yogurt, and there are some very good simple white cheeses such as ricotta and low-fat cottage cheese; although these are pasteurized they are low in fat and can be used as an adjunct to a biogenic salad or as part of another dish. It's best to stay away from the heavy, hard cheeses: not only are they fairly acidic, they are also very rich in fat.

Free-range eggs, particularly if they are fertilized, are themselves biogenic foods (especially when raw) and certainly have a part to play in the biogenic diet. However, they are also a very highly concentrated source of protein; indeed, they offer the highest utilization of protein of any food. You need to eat very few eggs to benefit from them.

Yogurt can be an extremely good food on the biogenic diet too – particularly if it is home-made (see pages 177–80 for instructions.) Sheep's yogurt is my favourite. Natural yogurt helps restore the healthy intestinal flora which have been damaged by eating a diet too high in refined foods or by taking antibiotics or other medication.

Dairy products of note are:

   butter (in small quantities and preferably salt free)
   cottage cheese   feta cheese
   other low-fat natural white
      cheeses such as Petit Suisse
   cows' yogurt   goats' yogurt
   sheep's yogurt   natural or unsweetened yogurt
   free-range eggs (preferably fertilized)

Flesh Foods

There is no necessity to eat flesh foods at all on the biogenic diet: you will get a full complement of proteins from the mixes of your sprouted seeds and grains, nuts, the occasional egg and low-fat cheese. However, if you do choose to eat flesh foods then they should be those foods which have had the least processing. This excludes most meats, such as beef, lamb and pork, since the flesh of these animals is very high in fat and also tends to contain a high level of biocidic contaminants which you want to avoid. So, if you choose to eat flesh foods, opt instead for free-range poultry, game and seafood (such as fish), all of which are lower in saturated fats and less likely to be contaminated. But remember that all flesh foods are highly concentrated and you certainly need not eat them more than two to three times a week.

One animal-food recipe worth remembering (and one of my own favourites) is Biogenic Omelette: stuff a plain omelette with whatever sprouts you have available, dressed with Light Vinaigrette, sprinkle the top with tamari (a kind of soy sauce), and serve.

Meat and fish vary tremendously in quality depending upon their freshness and on how much exposure the creatures have had to chemicals, growth hormones, artificial feeds and so forth. You can choose from:

free-range chicken	Cornish hens
fish	game
free-range turkey	seafood

Seasonings

Seasonings such as sea-salt, vegetable bouillon powder, tamari, herbs, spices and mustard have an important role to play in the biogenic diet. They bring great variety of taste to different sauces, soups, vegetable dishes and salads. Choose the very best of sauces and condiments, spices and herbs and use them in creative ways.

Sauces and Condiments

Honey

Raw honey is honey that has not been heated or thinned. It is rich in certain vitamins, minerals and enzymes, but is a very concentrated food and should therefore be used only in very small quantities.

Miso
A fermented soya-bean paste which is rich in digestive enzymes and high in protein. It can be used for seasoning soups and sauces. It is also a delicious addition to dips for crudités and salad dressings. See Resources for stockists.

Mustard
Either Dijon or Meaux.

Sea-salt
The only type of salt which you should use – and use it *sparingly*.

Tamari
A kind of naturally fermented soy sauce made by fermenting soya beans, wheat and sea-salt. It is a good seasoning for soups, salads and dressings.

Tahini
A paste made from ground sesame seeds which is delicious and very nutritious. It is a protein condiment.

Vegetable Bouillon Powder
An excellent natural seasoning made from vegetables, sea vegetables and sea-salt. It can be used in salad dressings, soups, vegetable dishes – I use it in very many of my recipes instead of salt. It is available from healthfood stores or direct from Marigold Health Foods Ltd, Unit 10, St Pancras Commercial Centre, 63 Pratt Street, London NW1 0BY.

Spices and Herbs
I grow many herbs in my own garden and use them constantly in my sauces, my soups and my salads. However, I also use packaged seasoning, particularly when the fresh herbs and spices are not available. Here are some herbs and spices that I strongly recommend for use in the biogenic diet:

allspice	cardamom
anise	caraway seeds
basil	cayenne
bay leaves	celery seeds

chervil
cinnamon
cloves
coriander
cumin seeds
curry powder
dill
fennel
ginger (preferably fresh)
lovage
mace
marjoram
mint

mustardseed
nutmeg
oregano
paprika
parsley
pepper (black)
rosemary
sage
summer savory
tarragon
thyme
turmeric
winter savory

Drinks

Juices If you are lucky enough to have your own centrifugal juice extractor (see pages 128–9) you can make some excellent drinks from vegetables and fruits – for instance, by mixing raw carrot juice and raw apple juice half and half. Building upon this formula you can add a little cucumber or mustard and cress or celery or fresh tomatoes to create some delicious biogenic cocktails.

Because these juices contain no fibre the vegetables and fruits mix very well with each other, and they will be absorbed within 15 to 20 minutes of drinking them. They make an excellent beginning to a biogenic meal.

If you are not fortunate enough to have a juice extractor you can buy some very good European vegetable and fruit juices which have been processed at low heat. 'Biotta' make several good kinds. In Britain 'Aspell' apple juice is a very good low-heat-processed natural apple juice.

Water Drink only water that has been filtered, in order to remove some of the chlorine and heavy metals it contains, or bottled spring water.

Tea and coffee These do not belong in the biogenic diet because both of them can leave large quantities of toxic residues in the system. Instead, try Café Hag (decaffeinated), some of the excellent coffee substitutes such as Lane's Dandelion Coffee, or Pioneer, or some of the excellent herb teas. I particularly like those made by 'Celestial Seasonings': my favourites are their Cinnamon and Rose, Sleepy-time, Red Zinger and Almond Sunset. You can add a teaspoonful of raw honey for sweetening if you want to.

21
Blissful Breakfast

BREAKFAST IS SHEER bliss. The easiest part of the biogenic diet, it consists of nothing but fruit. The reason for this is simple – as we saw on pages 132–3.

The digestion of fruit is so easy that it requires only a tiny fraction of the energy which is needed to break down other foods in your body. All fruits – except bananas, dates and dried fruit, which stay in your stomach for about 45 minutes or so – are in your stomach no more than 20 to 30 minutes. There they are broken down and rapidly release their vitamins and minerals, so that these nutrients are almost instantly made available for absorption into the bloodstream. And, because they require so little energy for digestion, the energy available to your body is not disturbed when you eat them but can continue to focus on the elimination processes which are central to the detoxification of your system and encourage fat-loss.

Eat Fruit Alone

The thing to remember about fruit is that, since it does not stay in the stomach for very long, it is best eaten on its own. It should certainly not be eaten together with other foods, such as protein foods or most starchy foods – although nuts and low-fat dairy products such as yogurt and cottage cheese can combine quite well with some fruits. (See the chart on pages 136–7.) Neither should you eat fruits immediately after a concentrated protein or starch food. However, when you eat them on an empty stomach – the best way for fruits to be eaten – their effect is extremely positive: they accelerate detoxification and encourage weight-loss.

Fruit has the highest water content of any food: between 75 per cent and 90 per cent of all fruit consists of natural mineral water. Raw fruit also contains a beneficent mix of ions (electro-magnetically charged particles): this mixture appears to be helpful in enhancing metabolic functions on a cellular level. This lends to fruit an ability to cleanse even long-standing residues from your tissues.

Man the Fruit-Eater

The digestive tract of man, like those of his close relatives the apes and other fruit-eating animals, is of length between 12 and 14 times the height of his body. By contrast, a grass-eater's digestive tract is more than 20 times its body-length, and carnivores have a digestive tract which is only about 5 times body-length. Anthropologists confirm that our early ancestors were not predominantly meat-eaters or even gatherers of seeds, shoots, leaves and grasses; neither do they appear to have been omnivorous. Instead they lived chiefly on a diet of fruit. This has been determined primarily by studying the striations, or markings, on the fossilized teeth of early specimens and by examining the contents of fossilized intestines. While no one could sensibly suggest that anyone today go on a totally fruit diet, fruit offers such an important tool in the biogenic programme for weight-loss that to ignore it would be to undermine your body's full potential for detoxification and fat metabolism.

That is why you begin each day with fruit. This can either be fruit in its simple, original form – an apple or two, fresh berries, apricots or melon – or it can entail using fruits to create delicious and even elaborate fruit dishes to delight your aesthetic senses. The practical advantages of eating fruits on their own are obvious. Breakfast takes almost no time at all and certainly no preparation if it consists of something as simple as a handful of apricots or a couple of figs, an apple or two or half a grapefruit. For most people this will suffice. But when you begin to explore the different delicious possibilities of dishes that can be made from fruit they can seem too tempting to resist preparing them – especially for beautiful Sunday breakfasts in bed!

Plain or fancy, whichever you choose, make sure that at least 20 per cent to 30 per cent of your daily fare comes in the form of fresh fruits. Try to eat a variety of fruits each week and choose your fruits, as much as possible, so that you eat them when they are in season. They will supply a major portion of the essential vitamins and minerals your body needs to function at a very high level of wellbeing.

Fruits – The Master Cleansers

It is not only because they require little digestion (so that the energy otherwise used to digest food can be used to continue the detoxification process) and because they help heighten the micro-electrical potentials of cell tissues that fruits are so efficient for cleansing the body. They are also good detoxifiers because they contain a high percentage of carbon. The high carbon content of fruits encourages them to act as incinerators of waste matter in the digestive system as well as in the bloodstream, the internal organs, the skin and, on a cellular level, elsewhere throughout your body.

Fresh fruits are also alkalinizing to the system – even the acid fruits. This is very important for your body for it can encourage cellular repair and help counteract the acidic wastes eliminated from the cells which tend to build up when you are under stress (in fact, most of the by-products of stress are acidic). Not just the raw fruits but also the biogenic foods and the other bioactive foods, such as fresh raw vegetables, help increase your resistance to stress and fatigue thanks to their ability to render the blood slightly more alkaline.

A few people claim that fresh fruit is difficult for them to digest. This should not be the case provided you never eat it *with* any other kind of food or *following* anything else. Occasionally someone will experience a sense of bloating and wind if they are not used to eating fresh fruits when, at first, they begin eating them for breakfast. This is because the fruits' powerful cleansing ability encourages rapid elimination of toxicity, and in the process can temporarily create wind and bloating (it can also be because of a severe *Candida albicans* infection). But this is not a common experience. When it does occur it usually clears up within a day or two.

Breakfast Starts Here

Every morning choose whatever fruit appeals to you and eat as much of it as you feel comfortable with. You need not worry about the calories that your fruit contains. Simply listen to your own 'inner voice' to tell you when you've had enough and stop there. And remember to do as Fletcher did (see page 75) – chew each bite of the fruit you eat thoroughly. This complete chewing is the only way you will derive the full benefit from whatever you're eating.

Above all *don't let yourself overeat* ... but don't let yourself undereat either. Eat enough fruit that you feel satisfied. Be pleased with what you're eating, enjoy it, and remember that the fruits you're eating are playing an important part in the detoxification process that will allow you to lose excess fat permanently. If in the middle of the morning you find that you feel hungry again, by all means have another piece of fruit – or even two. Remember, though, to leave at least 30 minutes after eating a piece of fruit before you begin your lunch.

The lists of fruits you can choose from is a long one – just look at the list on page 140. The dried fruits such as figs, peaches, coconut, pears, pineapple, prunes, apricots, raisins, sultanas and apples are too concentrated for slimmers (remember the 70 per cent rule): they are best left alone until you have achieved the desired fat-loss: then you can incorporate them into your diet.

If you wish you can turn your fruits into fresh fruit juices, although it is far better to take the fruit as a whole since the natural fibre in fruit also plays an important part in the detoxification process. A delightful way of getting the best of both worlds is to mix a particular fruit, say a mango, in a blender together with a little orange or apple juice. It makes an absolutely delicious fresh fruit frappé which you can either drink or make thick enough to eat with a spoon. Such a drink is a meal in itself – as are many of the fruit dishes you'll find on pages 163–72. They make delightful total-meal recipes which are particularly good for light suppers. Use them often. Meanwhile here are the important points about fruit breakfasts.

Guidelines for the Bioactive Breakfast
- Eat as much fruit as you like up to one pound at a time, but make sure that you chew it very thoroughly.

- If you are hungry in the middle of the morning have another piece or two of fruit.
- Steer clear of the dried fruits until you have eliminated all the excess fat you want to shed.
- Eat bananas only if you are very hungry and feel that you want a heavier food, and remember that they take longer to digest: allow 45 minutes after eating a banana before eating your lunch.
- *Never overeat* . . . but likewise never undereat. Eat just as much as you need to feel satisfied.

22
A Biogenic Fortnight

HERE IS AN outline of suggested menus to get you started. You will find the recipes in the chapters that follow (use the index) – except in the case of the flesh foods. I have given alternatives three or four days a week depending upon whether or not you want to eat the flesh foods. If you do, remember that the best ones are game, fish, seafood and free-range poultry. If you don't, then simply take the other option. Lunch and supper are interchangeable.

These menus are only guidelines to get you started. Play with them and create your own biogenic foodstyle around what you like best.

DAY ONE

Breakfast
Fresh fruit, either *au naturel* or made into a fruit frappé or fruit salad. Have as much as you like but chew it well so that you extract all the goodness and flavour from each bite. If you are hungry you may have another couple of pieces of fruit or a fruit drink mid-morning as well. Should you choose melon as your fruit, don't mix it with other fruits – eat it on its own.

Lunch
Sprouted Lentil Salad
and
Barley Mushroom Soup

Dinner
Green Glory Salad
Baked Leeks and Pecans
or
Grilled Chicken Breast with Lemon
Baked Parsnips

DAY TWO

Breakfast
Same as on day one

Lunch
Red Witch Salad
Yummy Brown Rice

Dinner
Bioactive Avocado and Tomato Soup
Mange-tout and Almond Stir-Fry
Mixed Green Side Salad with French Spice Dressing

DAY THREE

Breakfast
Same as on day one

Lunch
Fresh Orange Juice
(leave 20 minutes before main course)
Bulgar Salad with Endive

Dinner
Gazpacho
Easy Vegetable Curry
Small Sprout Salad with Italian Dressing

DAY FOUR

Breakfast
Same as on day one

Lunch
Green Light Salad
Racy Red Cheese
Avocado Delight Dressing

Dinner
Spicy Shish-Kebab
Kasha *or* Brown Rice
Sliced Tomatoes with Sprout Splendour Dressing

DAY FIVE

Breakfast
Same as on day one

Lunch
Baked Potato stuffed with Blue Dolphin Salad
Horsey Tomato Dressing
or
Snappy Apple Salad with Cottage Cheese

Dinner
Jerusalem Artichoke Salad
Light Vinaigrette Dressing
Aubergine Pâté
or
Poached salmon with fresh parsley and lemon juice
Baked Onion

DAY SIX

Breakfast
Same as on day one

Lunch
Celebration Salad
or
Pineapple Treasures Served with Nuts

Dinner
Biogenic Soup
Vegi-Stroganoff

DAY SEVEN

Breakfast
Same as on day one

Lunch
Spring Gardens Salad
Nut Mayonnaise *or* Pink Yogurt Dressing
or
Berry Muesli

Dinner
Tomato Treasures
Split Pea Soup
or
Braised Vegetables

DAY EIGHT

Breakfast
Same as on day one

Lunch
Greek Delight Plus Salad
or
Summer Red and White Fruit Salad

Dinner
Root-Is-Best Salad
Celery Special Dressing
Biogenic Omelette

DAY NINE

Breakfast
Same as on day one

Lunch
Large bowl of crudités served with
Soya Cottage Cheese, Tahini Mayonnaise
or Raw Houmus

Dinner
Watercress Salad
Italian Dressing
Biogenic Stir-Fry
Millet

DAY TEN

Breakfast
Same as on day one

Lunch
Corn Soup
Cress Special
Horsey Tomato Dressing

Dinner
Charismatic California Salad
(with a sweet Cashew Cream to which you
have added a tablespoonful of raw honey)
or
Ratatouille and Raita Salad

DAY ELEVEN

Breakfast
Same as on day one

Lunch
Courgette Tomato Soup
Branton's Booster
Light Vinaigrette *or* Italian Dressing

Dinner
Small Cress Special Salad
Barley Pilaff
Minty Peas

DAY TWELVE

Breakfast
Same as on day one

Lunch
Crudités served with
Potato Supreme Salad

Dinner
Sliced Cucumbers
Light Vinaigrette
Sesame Stir-Fry
Kasha

DAY THIRTEEN

Breakfast
Same as on day one

Lunch
Greek Delight Plus

Dinner
Slice of melon (don't forget the 20 minutes!)
Easy Vegetable Curry
Yummy Brown Rice *or* Millet

DAY FOURTEEN

Breakfast
Same as on day one

Lunch
Scottish Pine Salad

Dinner
Red Witch Salad
Curried Pumpkin Soup
or
Braised Vegetables
or
Prawns grilled in a little oil and garlic

Now that we've looked at some sample menus, let's explore the recipes themselves. We'll start with the fruit dishes, then look at how to grow your own sprouts, culture your own yogurt and make your own seed and nut dishes.

23
Fabulous Fruits

AMONG THE GREATEST pleasures of the biogenic diet are some of the beautiful fruit dishes you can prepare as total meals. An all-fruit meal is a wonderful way to end the day – an ideal light supper. Also, a fruit salad with a little fresh yogurt makes an energizing lunch, and I love making a quick fruit frappé instead of a meal in the middle of summer when everyone longs for something cool and frothy. In this chapter you will find some of my family's favourite fruit treats. Some are suitable for breakfast since they are made of fruit only; others are designed as lunch or dinner dishes.

These are only my personal inventions. Fruits offer such a wide range of colours, textures and flavours, and there are so many ways of using them, that you will no doubt create even more beautiful dishes on your own. When you do I would love to hear about them!

Remember that you can always start your lunch or dinner with a simple all-fruit appetizer such as a piece of cold melon or a bunch of sweet grapes, or a glass of freshly pressed fruit and vegetable juice. But, if you do, allow 20 to 30 minutes before beginning your next course.

In all the recipes used in this book, C = cupful, tbsp = tablespoonful, tsp = teaspoonful.

Summer Red-and-White Fruit Salad
A stunningly beautiful fruit salad which makes a luscious full-fruit meal.

1 C cherries, pitted and halved
1 C plums, pitted and quartered
1 C raspberries
outer leaves of a lettuce
12 oz low-fat cottage cheese
1/2 pineapple (outer skin cut off, flesh cut into rings, core removed)
1 tbsp finely chopped pineapple mint or apple mint

Combine the cherries, plums and raspberries and mix well. Arrange a few lettuce leaves on a plate and lay pineapple rings on top. Place a scoop of cottage cheese in the centre of the ring and pour the other fruit mixture over the top and sprinkle with fresh mint.

Spiked Apricot Suprême

Another delicious fruit meal – not a breakfast dish – is this delightful and spicy combination of apricots, coconut and cinnamon.

6–8 ripe apricots, pitted and cut into small pieces
1/4 tsp cinnamon
1/4 tsp allspice
1 tbsp raw honey

For the Sauce
3/4 C dried coconut
a little spring water
1 tsp honey
1 tsp fresh vanilla essence

Blend half of the chopped apricots in a blender to which you add the cinnamon, allspice and honey. Arrange the rest of the apricots in glass dishes and pour the apricot spice mixture over them. To make coconut cream mix the dried coconut (make sure you do not buy the kind that has sugar added to it) with enough spring water in a blender to get the consistency of heavy cream. Add the honey and vanilla essence and continue to mix. Spoon the coconut cream onto the apricot dish and serve immediately.

Tropical Delight

I have an absolute passion for tropical fruit – I think I could live on it! This is a particularly tasty combination of some of my favourites.

1 papaw, peeled, seeded and sliced
2 ripe bananas, sliced lengthways twice, then chopped into small pieces
1 mango, peeled and diced
¼ C apple juice
2 tbsp coconut flakes
dash of nutmeg

Put the fruits into a bowl. Add the apple juice (you may use concentrated apple juice with a little spring water added if you prefer) by pouring over the fruit. Serve immediately garnished with coconut flakes and sprinkled with nutmeg.

Charismatic California Salad

A sunshine spectacular of the acid fruits, with avocado used as a source of protein and essential fatty acids. You can make this salad in any size – small if you want a small snack meal or very large indeed to create a large and extremely filling fruit meal.

1 orange
1 satsuma or tangerine
1 pink grapefruit
1 ripe avocado
3 or 4 large leaves from the outside of a lettuce
1 tbsp lemon juice
a few strawberries (optional)

Peel, remove the seeds and section the citrus fruits and cut the segments into bite-size pieces. Peel and chop the avocado and strawberries (if desired) and mix together with the other fruits. Add lemon juice and toss gently. Line a bowl with lettuce leaves and place mixed salad in the centre. Serve immediately.

Poire Suprême

Who would ever have thought such a splendid dish could be concocted from the simple pear?

4 pears, cored and sliced thinly but not peeled
2 tbsp raw honey
juice of 2 lemons
3 drops of oil of peppermint
1/2 C blackcurrants

Place the thinly sliced pears in a dish. Combine the honey, lemon juice and oil of peppermint in a glass and mix well with a spoon. Pour over the pears. Chill in a refrigerator for 30 minutes, then garnish with blackcurrants and serve immediately.

Tropical Promise

A simple yet delicious dish which I enjoy when papaws are readily available.

2 bananas
2 small papaws, peeled and seeded
3 tbsp desiccated coconut flakes
2 tbsp raisins which have been soaked in water for a few hours

Slice bananas and papaws and arrange on a salad plate. Sprinkle with coconut flakes and raisins. Serve immediately.

Aaron's Delight

This is a favourite of my son Aaron who has been virtually raised on fruit and sprouts. In fact I think the majority of the foods he eats, one way or another, are fruits. It is a very filling dish which can be eaten for breakfast or later on as a fruit meal on its own, or with desiccated coconut sprinkled on top.

2 large ripe bananas
8 fresh dates
2 tbsp desiccated or fresh grated coconut (optional)

Put the fruit into a blender and purée until smooth. Pour into individual glass dishes. Sprinkle with fresh grated or desiccated coconut (if desired) and serve.

Snappy Apple Salad

This is a simple and pleasant fruit salad based upon apples and grapes. It can be served as a main meal either with nuts such as pecans, almonds or hazels and a scoop of low-fat cottage cheese or a dish of fresh yogurt. I particularly like it with sheep's yogurt as a light supper.

3 sweet apples, chopped
1 orange, peeled, sectioned and cut into bite-size pieces
1 satsuma or tangerine, peeled, sectioned and cut into bite-size pieces
1 C fresh green grapes
1/2 tsp allspice
pinch of cinnamon
4 oz nuts or low-fat cottage cheese or yogurt

Combine all the fruits and spices. Mix and allow to chill in a refrigerator for 15–30 minutes. Serve the fruit in a large flat dish and top with yogurt, low-fat cottage cheese or chopped nuts. Serve immediately.

Stuffed Avocado

Another unusual and delightful main meal. Avocados combine beautifully with the acid fruits and berries. This dish is a surprise treat to the palate.

1 orange
1/4 C each of blackberries or
  strawberries or raspberries or all three
1 avocado (stone removed), sliced in half
pinch of freshly grated nutmeg

Chop and mix all fruits together. Fill the avocado boats with the fruit mixture and sprinkle with nutmeg. (Half an avocado is enough for one person.)

Pandora's Persimmon

This is one of the simplest recipes of all with fruit – and one of the most delicious.

2 very ripe persimmons
3/4 C desiccated coconut
a little spring water
1 tsp honey
1 tsp pure vanilla essence

Peel the ripe persimmons and blend thoroughly in a blender or food processor. Pour into chilled dishes. Mix the desiccated coconut in a blender with sufficient spring water to get the consistency of thick cream before adding the honey and vanilla essence and blending in well. Spoon the coconut cream onto the persimmon.

Pineapple Treasures

The perfect dish for a splendid Sunday brunch. Pineapple Treasures not only look wonderful, their flavourful combination of succulent berries and fresh pineapple almost melts in your mouth.

1 ripe pineapple
1 ripe avocado
1 C fresh raspberries or *strawberries* or *blackberries* or *¹/₃ C of each*
a little honey (optional)
2 tbsp chopped fresh pineapple mint or *spearmint*
2–3 tbsp chopped almonds or *hazelnuts* or *cashews (optional)*

Cut the pineapple in two lengthwise, scoop out the insides, cutting the pineapple flesh into cubes. Toss it together with the other fresh fruits, including the avocado; you may add a little honey if you wish. Refill the pineapple shells with this fruit salad mixture and garnish with the mint. May be served for breakfast or as a main meal. As a main meal you can sprinkle with 2 to 3 tbsp of chopped almonds, hazelnuts or cashews.

Prune Whip

This is an excellent dish to make for breakfast or a fruit meal in the middle of winter when you have very little fresh fruit in the house. It can be made with either spring or filtered water or apple juice. You may even use apple-juice concentrate mixed with a little spring water if you like.

1 C dried prunes
1 C spring water or *filtered water* or *apple juice*
dash cinnamon
few slices of apple or pear (optional)

Soak dried prunes in apple juice or water to cover overnight. Remove stones and blend or liquefy in a food processor or blender with enough of the juice to make a thick sauce adding a pinch of cinnamon. Slice a few pieces of apple or pear to use as a garnish (if desired) and serve.

Live Apple Sauce

The quality and taste of this apple sauce depend entirely upon the quality of the apples themselves. If you make it with beautiful red apples it turns out to be a gorgeous pink colour. It is a real favourite for children and makes a lovely fruit breakfast or, served with 4 oz chopped pecans, can be an excellent fruit meal for later on in the day.

4 apples, cored but not peeled and cut into small pieces
¾ C (more or less) of apple juice
dash of cinnamon or nutmeg or caraway or aniseed
a little raw honey (optional)

Liquefy the chopped apples in enough apple juice to make a medium-thick sauce. Add spices and a little raw honey to sweeten if desired. Serve immediately, lightly sprinkled with cinnamon, nutmeg, caraway or aniseed.

Almond Apple Porridge

Apples, with their remarkable ability to combine well with all sorts of foods which you wouldn't expect, make a wonderful marriage with almonds. Not a breakfast dish, because of the nuts it contains, this recipe nonetheless makes a yummy fruit meal for later on in the day.

4 apples, cored and cut into pieces but not peeled
¼ C finely chopped almonds
juice of 1 lemon
juice of 1 orange
sprinkling of nutmeg

Blend the apples with the other ingredients, keeping aside 1 tsp of the almonds and the nutmeg. When the mixture is fully blended, pour into four dishes and sprinkle with the remaining almonds and the nutmeg. Serve immediately.

Well-Combined Mueslis

To encourage fat-loss it's best for the moment to steer clear of the traditional Birchermuesli because, for some people, the combinations of milk products and grains – even though the grains have been soaked to break their sugars down into more simple ones – can be difficult for many slimmers to handle. Therefore it's a good idea to learn to make mixed fruit mueslis. Once you've lost all the extra fat you want to lose and your system has rebalanced itself, then you can indulge in the pleasures of the traditional Birchermuesli. In the meantime the suggestions below more than make up for what you think you're missing.

Berry Muesli

5–7 oz berries (strawberries, blackberries, blackcurrants, raspberries, etc.)
1 banana
1 tbsp finely chopped almonds or *pecans* or *cashews*
dash of cinnamon

Crush the berries with a fork. Slice the banana. Sprinkle with finely chopped almonds, pecans or cashews. Add a dash of cinnamon and serve immediately.

Other Mixed Fruit Muesli Suggestions

Blackberries and apples
Apples and sultanas
Apples and oranges
Apples and bananas
Plums, peaches and apricots
Strawberries and apples
Blueberries and apples

In each case remove the stones of any stoned fruit and blend in a food processor or chop finely with a knife. Otherwise the instructions are as for Berry Muesli.

Pear Surprise

Another delicious fruit-and-nut dish. Not suitable for breakfast but excellent if you desire a fruit meal later on in the day.

4 pears, finely grated
¹/₂ C raw cashews, ground

Fill four sorbet glasses with the finely grated pears and sprinkle each with the ground cashews. Serve immediately.

Fruit Drinks that Make a Meal

Apricot Lhassi

A fresh fruit frappé with a delightful Eastern flavour.

4–5 fresh apricots, stones removed
juice of 2 small oranges
pinch of coriander

Put the ingredients into a blender and blend thoroughly. You may add ice if you wish to make a delicious cold summer breakfast.

Apple Raspberry Frappé

2 sweet apples, cored but not peeled, cut into small pieces
¹/₂ tsp finely chopped lemon balm or mint
¹/₂ C fresh or frozen raspberries
spring or filtered water (optional)
ice cubes (optional)

Place the ingredients in a blender and liquidize, adding a little spring or filtered water to thin it if you wish, and ice cubes if you want a chilled dish.

Pineapple Blackberry Frappé

2 C fresh pineapple chunks
¹/₂ C blackberries
juice of ¹/₂ a lime (optional)
spring or filtered water (optional)
ice cubes (optional)

Place all the ingredients into a blender and liquidize. This can be thinned using a little spring or filtered water and chilled with an ice cube or two.

Strawberry Cream Shake

Not a breakfast recipe. This shake is a full fruit meal in itself and makes a lovely light supper for hot summer evenings.

½ C fresh cashews
1 C spring or filtered water
½ C strawberries
1 tbsp raw honey
½ C fresh pineapple chunks (optional)

Blend all the ingredients (including the pineapple chunks, if desired) in a food processor or blender and serve in a tall frosted glass. This makes one very large shake.

Banana-Coconut-Mint Frappé

Another full fruit meal which is rich and creamy.

2 very ripe bananas
¼ C desiccated or shredded fresh coconut
1 tsp freshly chopped mint leaves
ice cubes (optional)

Blend ingredients together in a food processor or blender and serve. You may add one or two ice cubes to chill.

Creamy Date Delight

2 very ripe bananas
4 fresh dates
1 tbsp shredded coconut
½–1 C sparkling spring water

Blend the bananas, dates and coconut together thoroughly in a blender or food processor, then add the sparkling water and mix gently. Pour into chilled glasses and serve immediately.

24
The Home-Mades

TO ME, NOTHING surpasses the best of home-made food. And there are three kinds of foods in the biogenic diet which are particularly good when you do it all yourself: sprouts, yogurt and the lovely seed milks, creams and cheeses. They are also so simple to make that it seems a shame to buy them. We'll look at all three in turn.

How to Sprout
The most important staple of the biogenic diet, sprouts are easy to grow any time and just about anywhere. All you need to start your own indoor germinating 'factory' are a few old jars, some pure water, fresh seeds/grains/pulses, and an area of your kitchen or a windowsill which is not absolutely freezing. Sprouts form the basis of biogenic salads, soups and dressings. Most sprouts are neutral foods and can combine with either proteins or starches.

Home-Made Sprouters
There are two main ways to sprout seeds – in jars and in seed trays. Let's look at the traditional way first, then at the way I find easiest and best.

A simple and cheap sprouter can be anything from a bucket to a polythene bag. The traditional sprouter is a wide-mouthed glass jar. Some people like to make it all neat by covering the jar with a cheesecloth or a nylon or wire mesh and securing it with a rubber band, or using a mason jar with a screw-on rim to keep the cheesecloth in place. But I find the easiest and least fussy way is simply to use open jars and to cover a row of them with a tea towel to prevent dust and insects from getting in.

To Begin

- Put the seed/grain/pulse of your choice, for example mung, in a large sieve. (For amount to use see the chart on pages 186–7 and remember that most sprouts give a volume about eight times that of the dry seeds/grains/pulses.) Remove any small stones, broken seeds or loose husks and rinse your seeds well.
- Put the seeds in a jar and cover with a few inches of pure water. Rinsing can be done in tap water, but the initial soak, where the seeds absorb a lot of water to set their enzymes in action, is best done in spring, filtered or boiled and then cooled water, as the chlorine in tap water can inhibit germination – and is also not very good for you.
- Leave your seeds to soak overnight, or as long as is needed (see chart on pages 186–7).
- Pour off the soak-water – if none remains then you still have thirsty beans on your hands, so give them more water to absorb. The soak-water is good for watering houseplants. Some people like to use it in soups or drink it straight, but I find it extremely bitter. Also, the soak-water from some beans and grains contains phytates – nature's insecticides, which protect the vulnerable seeds in the soil from invasion by micro-organisms. These phytates interfere with certain biological functions in man including the absorption of many minerals (including zinc, magnesium and calcium), and are therefore best avoided. The soak-water from wheat, however, known as 'rejuvelac', makes a wonderful liquid for preparing fermented cheese and is very good for you.
- Rinse the seeds either by pouring water through the cheesecloth top, swilling it around and pouring it off several times, or by tipping the seeds of the open-topped jars into a large sieve and rinsing them well under the tap before replacing them in the jar. Be sure that they are well drained either way as too much water may cause them to rot. The cheesecloth-covered jars can be left tilted in a dish drainer to allow all the water to run out. Repeat

this morning and night for most sprouts. During a very hot spell they may need a midday rinse too.

- Return sprouter to a reasonably warm place. This can be under the sink, in an airing cupboard or just in a corner not too far from a radiator. Sprouts grow fastest and best without light and in a temperature of about 21°C (70°F).
- After about 3–5 days your sprouts will be ready for a dose of chlorophyll if you want to give them one. Alfalfa thrive on a little sunlight after they've grown for two or three days but mung beans, fenugreek and lentils are best off without it. Place alfalfa in the sunshine – a sunny windowsill is ideal – and watch them develop little green leaves. Be sure that they are kept moist and that they don't get too hot and roast!
- After a few hours in the sun most sprouts are ready to be eaten. Optimum vitamin content occurs 50–96 hours after germination begins. (See chart on pages 186–7 for specific growth times.) They should be rinsed and eaten straight away or stored in the refrigerator in an airtight container or sealed polythene bag. Some people dislike the taste of seed hulls such as those that come with mung sprouts. To remove them simply place the sprouts in a bowl and cover with water. Stir the sprouts gently. The seed hulls will float to the top and can be skimmed off with your hand. I personally don't mind the taste at all and prefer to eat the whole sprouts as the seed hulls are an excellent source of fibre.

Mass Production

Now for my favourite and simplified method using seed trays. I find that, with the great demand of my family for biogenic foods, the jar method simply doesn't produce enough. Also, for sprouted seeds, you have to rinse twice a day while tray sprouts need only a splash of water each day. Here is a very simple way to grow even very large quantities easily.

Take a few small seed trays (the kind gardeners use to grow seedlings, with fine holes in the bottom for drainage). When germinating very tiny seeds such as alfalfa you will need to line your seed tray with damp, plain white kitchen towels. For larger seeds the trays themselves are enough. Place the trays in a larger tray to catch the water that drains from them. Soak the seeds/grains/ pulses overnight as in the jar method, then rinse them well and spread them a few layers deep in each of the trays. Spray the seeds with water (by putting them under the tap or by using a spray bottle) and leave in a warm place. Check the seeds each day and spray them again if they seem dry. If the seeds get too wet they will rot, so be careful not to overwater them. Larger seeds such as chickpeas, lentils and mung beans need to be gently turned over with your hand once a day to ensure that the seeds underneath are not suffocated. Alfalfa seeds can be simply sprinkled and left alone and after four or five days will have grown into a thick green carpet. Don't forget to put the sprouts in some sunlight for a day or so to develop lots of chlorophyll. When the seeds are ready, harvest them, rinse them well in a sieve and put them in an airtight container or sealed polythene bag until you want them. To make the next batch, rinse the trays well and begin again.

Tips
Some sprouts are more difficult to grow than others, but usually if seeds fail to germinate at all it is because they are too old and no longer viable. It is always worth buying top-quality seeds because, after removing dead and broken seeds, and taking germinating failures into account, they work out better value than cheaper ones. Also try to avoid seeds treated with insecticide-fungicide mixtures such as those which are sold in gardening shops and some nurseries. Healthfood shops and wholefood emporiums are usually your best bet. At wholefood emporiums you can buy seeds very cheaply for sprouting in bulk. It is fun to experiment with growing all kinds of sprouts from radish seeds to soya beans, but avoid plants whose greens are known to be poisonous such as the deadly nightshade family, potato and tomato seeds. Also avoid kidney beans as they are poisonous raw.

Some of the easiest to begin with are alfalfa seeds, adzuki (aduki) beans, mung beans, lentils, fenugreek seeds, radish seeds, chick-peas and wheat. Others include sunflower seeds, pumpkin seeds, sesame seeds, buckwheat, flax, mint, red clover, peas, peanuts, almonds, triticale, rye, oats, sweetcorn (maize) and millet. These latter can sometimes be difficult to find or to sprout – the 'seeds' must be in their hulls and the nuts must be really fresh and undamaged.

Good luck!

Easy Yogurt-Making

As a health-giving protein food, yogurt is most important for its action on the intestinal flora. The lactic-acid bacteria it contains synthesize B vitamins, which are needed in the intestines. The acid medium they create in the colon is unfavourable for the growth of pathogenic and putrefactive bacteria. In fact, laboratory studies show that many pathogens, such as those causing typhoid fever, dysentery and diphtheria lose their virulence when placed in yogurt and are killed even in yogurt whey. This is one of the reasons why yogurt is very good for curing gastro-intestinal disorders. It is also useful in restoring the digestive tract after the use of antibiotics, which destroy all the intestinal bacteria (including the friendly ones) plus many of the B vitamins.

Yogurt is much more easily digested than milk. One reason is that the milk protein in it has been partially broken down by the bacteria. Perhaps even more important is the breakdown of lactose (milk sugar) to lactic acid which occurs when milk is made into yogurt. This is of significance because many people (whether they know it or not) have difficulty digesting this sugar. In adulthood they lose the ability to produce the enzyme lactase so that they can no longer break down lactose; this results in lactose intolerance. Undigested lactose remains in the intestines and attracts water. It can cause bloating and excessive flatulence as well as abdominal pains and diarrhoea. But many people who experience difficulties with drinking milk can eat yogurt without any problem. Another advantage to yogurt is that the calcium and phosphorus contained in it are much more available for absorption than in milk.

The best yogurt is made from sheep's or goats' milk. Cows' milk is harder to digest and more mucus-forming. Goats' and sheep's milk and yogurt can be bought at healthfood shops while plain natural cows' milk yogurt can be found in supermarkets.

Making Your Own Yogurt

Yogurt-making is really a lot easier than most people think. You don't need fancy yogurt-makers, thermometers, sterilizing fluids, etc. All you need is some milk, a container, a warm place and a 'starter'.

It is really worthwhile to try making your own yogurt because, provided you can get good fresh goats' or sheep's milk to make it from – or even powdered skimmed cows' milk – it needn't be heated above body-temperature, and so you retain the health-giving enzymes in the milk. Also, home-made yogurt is so much better-tasting than bought. One reason is that manufactured yogurt is not as fresh as it could be. It also sometimes contains stabilizers and preservatives which prevent it from spoiling too quickly. The result is a slightly tangy sour taste which can put people off yogurt. The natural home-made kind is actually sweet-tasting. With a little practice you can very quickly become an expert at making it.

Milk
Goats' and sheep's milk are best. You can buy a large quantity frozen and keep it in your freezer if you have the space. Soya milk can also be used (though take care – most soya milk is packed in aluminium cartons from which the soya bean, being acid, leaches the metal. See Resources for stockists of soya milk in non-aluminium cartons.) If you want to make cows' milk yogurt you can use low-fat skimmed milk powder. This is slightly better than whole milk and is very simple to use as it does not need to be boiled.

Container Use whatever you happen to have as a container. An earthenware pot, crock or casserole, heat-resistant wide-mouthed glass jar, wide-mouthed thermos flask or a stainless-steel cooking pot will do. Whatever you choose, it should be made of an inert material: no aluminium or flaky lacquered dishes. The container should have a lid.

A warm place
There are many ways of getting round this one. Country stoves such as Agas are ideal. The container can be stood directly on an upside-down saucer or a wire cooling tray on top if the stove is too hot. An airing cupboard or an oven heated to 120°F (50°C) and then switched off are both good. If you choose a radiator, or the warm area at the top back of the fridge, the container should be wrapped

in a blanket or towel for insulation. You can also use a polystyrene bucket or picnic hamper with a lid to make an 'incubator', or even make a simple 'hay box' using a couple of cardboard boxes: one is used as a lid to fit over the other with the yogurt container in the centre surrounded by blanket/hay/newspaper or any insulating material. The ideal temperature to be maintained is 90–105°F (32–40°C). You can also use a wide-mouthed thermos which will retain the blood heat you need to culture the yogurt for 6 to 8 hours and is ideal.

Starter
There are two kinds of starter – plain yogurt or powdered culture (the latter can be found in some healthfood shops). The yogurt starter can be of any sort of milk (cows' milk if you can't get hold of goats' or sheep's). It should be plain, natural yogurt with nothing added. Read labels! Some things advertised as yogurt in supermarkets in fact contain no lacto-bacteria at all. And don't buy fruit yogurt: it doesn't work and it also contains sugar. Once you make your first batch of yogurt you can use your own yogurt as a starter indefinitely. In fact the yogurt gets tastier each time you do. If it starts to become sour then use a fresh starter.

To Make about Two Pints of Yogurt
- Heat two pints (1 litre) of milk to just below boiling point (small bubbles should just be appearing at the edges of the pan). You can buy a round china disc that goes in the bottom of the pan and begins to rattle at the point when you need to remove the milk from the heat. (If you're using fresh goats' or sheep's milk from a good supplier, you can skip this step and just warm the milk to body temperature.)
- Leave the milk to cool to the temperature where you can comfortably put a finger into it and keep it there. It should feel neither hot nor cold – about blood-heat.
- Rinse your container with boiling water. This sterilizes it, which is important because you don't want any foreign bacteria in your yogurt. It also warms it and helps keep the milk at a constant temperature while the yogurt is incubating.
- Pour the milk into the container and add your culture. You will

need a generous tablespoonful of yogurt for each pint of milk you use. If you are using milk powder, mix it with pure blood-heat water in a blender – the more powder you use, the thicker your yogurt will be – then add your starter.

- Stir the culture in well. This is important to distribute the bacteria – otherwise you can end up with a lump of yogurt swimming in a dish of milk. (Be sure that whatever you use to stir the mixture has been rinsed in hot water too.)
- Place the lid on the container, or cover with cling film (the yogurt bacteria are anaerobic). Put the container into a warm place and leave for about 6 to 8 hours. The faster the yogurt curdles, the sweeter it will be. If it hasn't cultured in this time (it can take up to 10 hours), leave it longer.

Goats' and sheep's milk yogurts tend to be thinner than cows' milk ones. If you get a rather watery yogurt first time, don't worry: it is still delicious and it tends to get thicker each time a new batch is cultured. Experiment with the temperature of the warm place. Yogurt keeps in the refrigerator for up to about a week. Use it with fruit to make delicious yogurt drinks, or for soups and salad dressings.

Seed and Nut Milks, Creams and Butters

These are protein-based recipes. A simple seed milk can form an interesting protein-based meal on its own or it can be mixed with the acid fruits such as blackberries, raspberries, satsumas, pineapple, strawberries, plums and oranges, and even a few of the sub-acid fruits, such as apples, apricots, peaches, pears and sweet cherries, in order to make delicious protein-based fruit drinks – again, full meals in themselves.

The nut creams can be used in a number of interesting ways. You can either use them as toppings for fruit salads made from acid fruits and sub-acid fruits, in which case they are served in their 'sweet' form, or you can mix them with savoury herbs, seasoning (such as vegetable bouillon powder), spices, garlic, etc., in order to create interesting toppings for cooked vegetables, dips for crudités and, in a slightly thinned form, interesting salad dressings.

Nut butters are delicious used as spreads on raw vegetables such as sliced cucumbers or sliced carrot rounds. They are also good added to soups to give them a creamy texture and flavour.

Seed and Nut Milks

Almond Milk

Easy to digest, this milk is an excellent drink. It can be mixed together with apple juice or carrot juice (if you have a juice extractor) instead of water to make a delicious, easy-to-assimilate protein meal.

½ C almonds
2 tsp raw honey or *a few small stoned dates*
2 C spring or *filtered water*
½ tsp pure vanilla essence (optional)

Blanch the nuts by pouring boiling water over them and allowing them to sit for a minute or two. Then rub them between your fingers to remove the brown skins. Don't allow the nuts to remain in the water, however, for they will become waterlogged. Dry the nuts and grind very finely in a food processor or blender, then add the water and continue to mix until the mixture becomes a very fine paste. Add the honey and mix in thoroughly. You can add ½ tsp of pure vanilla essence if you like, or a few small stoned dates in place of the honey.

Variations on the Almond Milk theme You can use apple juice instead of water for an apple/almond milk drink. You can use half carrot juice and half water for a delicious carrot/almond milk.

Cashew Milk

This is a particularly light and bland nut milk. A favourite of children.

½ C cashews
1 C spring or *filtered water*
dash of cinnamon or *nutmeg*

Blend all the ingredients together in a food processor or blender for two minutes, adding extra water if necessary.

Sunflower-Seed Milk

An excellent source of high-quality protein, sunflower-seed milk can be added to soups or drunk as a sweet drink.

1 C sunflower seeds, finely ground
2 C spring or filtered water
*1/2 tsp pure vanilla essence or seasoning and herbs (see
    text)*
1 tbsp currants (optional)

Blend the ingredients together thoroughly in a blender or food processor, adding more water if necessary. For a savoury sunflower-seed milk replace the vanilla by 1 tsp of vegetable bouillon powder and add whatever fresh herbs are at hand, such as parsley, lovage or fresh basil. Curry powder is also a pleasant addition to sunflower-seed milk, as are allspice and cardamom.

Pine-Kernel Milk

An extremely rich, yet smooth and digestible vegetable-protein drink.

3 tbsp pine kernels
1 1/2 C filtered or spring water
1 tsp raw honey

Prepare as sunflower-seed milk.

Sesame Milk

A delicious seed milk with an Eastern flavour.

1/2 C sesame seeds
1 1/2 C spring or filtered water
2 tsp raw honey

Blend thoroughly in a food processor or blender, as for the other seed and nut milks.

Carob Milk

This is a particularly delicious chocolatey drink made from the carob fruit.

¹/₂ C cashews
³/₄ C spring or filtered water
3 tsp carob flour
1 tsp pure vanilla essence
1 tsp raw honey or a few dates

Blend all the ingredients together in a blender or food processor, adding more water if necessary.

Nut and Seed Butters and Creams
You can make excellent nut butters from raw nuts such as almonds, pecans, brazils, cashews, hazels or black walnuts by putting the nuts into a food processor or blender and blending them until they turn into a paste.

In the case of almonds you will probably need to add a little vegetable oil because they are harder than most nuts and therefore do not become as creamy. This oil can be corn oil, sesame oil or sunflower-seed oil, and you add it according to the texture as you're grinding the nuts to get just the right smoothness.

1¹/₂ C nuts
1–4 tbsp vegetable oil depending upon the kind of nuts you are using (some nuts need none)
¹/₂ tsp vegetable bouillon powder or tamari or a pinch of sea-salt

Put the oil into the food processor or blender and add the nuts slowly, blending until they become either smooth or crunchy depending upon the consistency you want. Keep scraping away the mixture from the side of the food processor to ensure that the entire mixture becomes blended well. Refrigerate after making.

These nut butters make excellent additions to soups. You use them the way you would use a tablespoon or two of cream by adding them just before the soup is served. Thinned slightly they also offer very pleasant dips for crudités.

Nut and Seed Cheeses
These cheeses are, in texture, between the nut and seed milks and the nut and seed butters. They are a particularly pleasant contrast to the freshness of salads and are excellent served together with crudités, salads or other raw dishes.

They come in two varieties – fermented and unfermented. Fermented seed and nut cheeses take about 6 to 12 hours to culture, depending upon the temperature of the room they are sitting in. They have a delightful sweet and tangy taste all their own.

The fermentation process helps break down the protein and therefore renders these seed and nut cheeses very digestible. Fermented foods are not only delicious, they are valuable to health. Rich in enzymes and in helpful bacteria, the proteins they contain are 'predigested' and therefore very easy for your body to assimilate. The lactic acid present in ferments destroys harmful intestinal bacteria, while the ferments themselves help your digestion, intestinal vitamin production, and the assimilation of nutrients.

You can also eat seed and nut cheeses which have not been fermented, in which case the taste is lighter. In our family, because seed and nut cheeses are so popular, it is difficult to allow them to sit for the eight hours or so necessary for the fermentation process to take place, so they are usually eaten fresh after they are made.

You can make a seed and nut cheese from almost any seed/nut combination. Here is the basic recipe.

1 C nuts and/or seeds
1 C spring or *filtered water* or *rejuvelac* (see page 185)
1 tsp vegetable bouillon powder or *1 tbsp tamari*
fresh herbs such as parsley, mint, lovage, marjoram, chives, basil (whatever you happen to have)

Grind the nuts and/or seeds as finely as possible in a food processor or blender. Add the water, herbs and seasoning and mix well until it is a fine paste, adding more water if necessary. Put the mixture into a bowl, cover with a tea towel and put in a warm place for eight hours or overnight. A warming cupboard is an excellent place to do this.

You can also add a couple of tablespoonfuls of white wine, some curry powder or some garlic to seed and nut cheeses. Some of the best combinations are: cashew on its own; sunflower and cashew; sunflower and sesame; and pesto (which is made from pine kernels and fresh basil leaves plus a little oregano, ½ C olive oil and garlic). Almond cheese is particularly good seasoned with a little curry powder. Brazil and cashew nuts and hazelnuts on their own are good choices.

Rejuvelac

Rejuvelac is simply the fermented soak-water from wheat sprouts. It is used to make seed and nut cheeses and other ferments. It can be drunk straight to clean the system and to improve the condition of intestinal flora.

Rejuvelac contains eight B vitamins as well as vitamins E and K. Its protein and carbohydrates are broken down into component amino acids and simple sugars respectively, so its nutrients are readily assimilated.

How To Make It

Soak a cup of wheat grains in about three cups of pure water for two days. Pour off the soak-water (rejuvelac) and use or refrigerate. Add another two cups of water to the grains and leave for a day. Again pour off the rejuvelac and refrigerate or use. This can be repeated for about three days after the initial 48-hour soak. At the end of this time the wheat berries can be eaten. Rejuvelac should taste quite sweet, not sour or tart. If it tastes unpleasant, it has probably been over-fermented. Rejuvelac will keep in the refrigerator for up to five days.

Sprouting Chart

Variety	Soak Time	Dry Measure (for litre)	Size at Harvest	Days to Harvest	Sprouting Tips	Nutritional Highlights	Suggested Uses
Adzuki (aduki)	Overnight	1 C	1 in	3–5	Sprout easily; good short or long	Rich in protein, iron, calcium. Benefits kidneys especially	Salads, oriental dishes, sandwiches, casseroles
Alfalfa	Overnight	3 tbsp	1–1½ in	4–5	Grow on wet paper towel; place in light last 24 hours to develop chlorophyll	Complete protein; vitamins A, B, C, D, E, F, K; rich in iron and phosphorus; alkaline	Salads, sandwiches, juices, soups, dressings
Almond	Overnight	2 C	Same	1	Swells but does not sprout	Rich in protein, calcium, fats	Salads, cereals, dressings, dips, sauces
Chickpea	Up to 24 hours	2 C	1 in	3–4	Needs long soak; renew water twice during soak	Complete protein; good provider of minerals	Dips, spreads, casseroles, salads, breads; good mixed with lentils or wheat
Fenugreek	Overnight	½ C	½–1 in	3–5	Pungent flavour	Rich in iron, vitamin A, protein; good detoxifier	Soups, curries, salads, loaves, casseroles; good mixed with other sprouts
Lentil	Overnight	1 C	½–1 in	3–5	Earthy flavour	Rich in B vitamins, protein (with grains), minerals; good source of fibre	Salads, soups, loaves, spreads, casseroles, curries

Millet	Overnight	1 C	¼ in	2–3	Use unhulled grains	Vitamins A and B, protein, fibre	Salads, breads, cereals, soups, casseroles
Mung	Overnight – at least	¾ C	½–1½ in	3–5	Grow in the dark for sweetness; last 24 hours in light	Complete protein; vitamins A, B and C, many minerals	Oriental dishes, soups, juices, sandwiches, salads
Mustardseed	Overnight	3 tbsp	½ in	4–5	Grow on damp cloth or paper towel; harvest the shoots	Minerals; a good tonic	Salads (excellent mixed with other sprouts), dressings
Radish	Do not soak	3 tbsp	1 in	4–5		Helps clear mucus and repair mucous membrane	Salads (mixes especially well with alfalfa), dressings, dips
Sesame	Overnight	3 C	Same	1–2	Keep growing-time brief as it can go bitter after 2 days	Calcium, vitamin E	Salads (mixes well with other small sprouts), dips, dressings
Sunflower	Overnight	3 C	Same	1–2	For best results make only what you need and eat fresh	Nutritionally best eaten on same day	Salads, soups, snacks, dips
Wheat and oats	Overnight	3 C	Same	2–3	Keep the soak-water of wheat (rejuvelac)	B vitamins, protein, fibre	Breads, soups, casseroles

25
Supersalads

TO MOST PEOPLE a salad is a pleasant side-dish you use to set off the main course – which is usually meat-based. On the biogenic diet everything is turned around. All the salads you will find in this section are meals in their own right. They can be served on their own for lunch or dinner or they can be combined with protein or starch side-dishes – soups, cheeses, breads, grain dishes, fish, chicken, egg dishes or game. They can also be made in much smaller quantities as side-salads to go with cooked main courses.

A biogenic salad is one in which the main ingredients are drawn from the biogenic sprouted seeds, grains and pulses. The other recipes are for bioactive salads based on fresh vegetables (there are also bioactive fruit salads such as those in Chapter 23). And finally of course there are the crudités, which make wonderful starters for a meal or, served in greater quantity with a rich dip, dressing or seed cheese, can themselves become a beautiful meal.

The salads here are mostly quite elaborate and mostly meant to be eaten as the centre of a meal. But you can also make some delightful, simple salads by taking a root vegetable, such as a grated turnip, carrot or parsnip, and combining it in equal amounts with both a leafy vegetable, such as watercress, lamb's lettuce or Chinese leaf, and a bulb vegetable such as red or green pepper. This is the classic formula for the simple salad and it works every time served with a beautiful dressing (see Chapter 26 for recipes). It is hard to go wrong following this principle, so experiment for yourself.

Biogenic Salads

The biogenic salad is the epitome of nutritional quality for encouraging fat-loss. It is made from the freshest and tastiest vegetables and sprouted seeds and grains that you can buy – or, far better, grow yourself. Make sure when you are choosing such things as cucumbers, celery and sweet peppers that they are firm and fresh and also that your carrots and broccoli are snappy and crisp.

Biogenic salads can be made either by hand (in which case the vegetables are cut with a sharp knife or grated on a stainless-steel hand grater) or in a food processor. All the ingredients in a biogenic salad are cut into bite-size pieces, except for lettuces and greens which are left in larger pieces to form a bed for the sprouts.

You can turn most of these salads into a protein meal by adding a seed cheese or a protein-based dip or salad dressing. You can turn them into a starch meal by eating them with a good wholegrain bread – preferably rye or pumpernickel, since the gluten in wheat tends to clog the intestines and may interfere with the elimination process – or serving them with wholegrain Scottish oatcakes, wholegrain crispbread or other wholegrain crackers.

You should treat the recipes listed below only as guidelines. The real pleasure of biogenic cuisine is creating masterpieces of your own out of the simple things which you grow yourself on your windowsill or find in your refrigerator.

Red Witch Salad (neutral)

The combination of radicchio with lamb's lettuce creates one of my favourite biogenic salads.

4 oz radicchio (Italian red lettuce) divided into leaves
2 oz lamb's lettuce
3 sticks of celery, chopped
2 large carrots, grated
1 C fresh mung-bean sprouts
3 oz chicory, divided into leaves
1 avocado, peeled and sliced
4 spring onions, chopped finely

For the Dressing
1 tbsp virgin olive oil
1 tbsp lemon or lime juice
1 tsp Meaux mustard

2 tsp chopped fresh basil
black pepper

Keeping out eight radicchio leaves and five leaves of chicory, mix all the salad ingredients together in a bowl. Then mix the ingredients for the dressing together in a screw-top jar by shaking well. Pour the dressing over the salad and toss. Now arrange the radicchio and chicory leaves which you have saved in a 'sunburst' around a platter. Serve the rest of the salad in the middle of the leaves.

Sprouted Lentil Salad (neutral)

This salad is a way of transforming the humble lentil into something quite marvellous.

1½ C fresh lentil sprouts
1 large red pepper (seeds removed), diced
4 oz broccoli florets
4 oz cauliflower florets
6 oz button mushrooms, sliced finely

For the Dressing
2 tbsp sesame oil
2 tbsp cider vinegar
1 tbsp freshly grated root ginger
2 tbsp fresh orange juice
1 tsp vegetable bouillon powder or soy sauce

Mix the salad ingredients together in a large bowl. Mix the dressing ingredients together in a screw-top jar and shake well. Pour the dressing over the salad and toss. You may garnish this salad with ¼ C of sunflower seeds if you like; this turns it into a protein salad.

A Touch of the Orient (neutral)

This salad has a typically oriental flavour and feel to it. It is pleasant served with slivers of blanched almonds, in which case it turns into a protein meal.

1 C mung-bean sprouts
1 C fenugreek sprouts
1 C adzuki sprouts

1 yellow or *red pepper, seeded and chopped*
1 medium carrot, chopped into ¹/₂ *in cubes*
¹/₂ C Chinese leaves, shredded finely
2 tbsp chopped fresh parsley
2 cloves of garlic, chopped very finely
¹/₄ C chopped spring onions
1 C spring or *filtered water*
juice of lemon
3 tbsp tamari
1 avocado, chopped into small cubes
the outside leaves of a cos lettuce

Marinate the sprouts and vegetables (except for the avocado and the cos leaves) in the water, to which you've added the lemon juice and tamari. Put in the refrigerator to chill. Then pour off the water and serve with small cubes of avocado on a bed of cos lettuce leaves, with or without a dressing.

Blue Dolphin Salad (neutral)

This simple biogenic salad can be completely transformed in quality depending upon the kind of dressing you serve it with. Experiment with a seed cheese, a good mayonnaise or a light Italian herbal dressing to see which you like best.

1 C lentil sprouts
1 C fenugreek sprouts
1 C alfalfa sprouts
1 C Chinese leaves, shredded finely
3 carrots, sliced in paper-thin rounds
1 avocado, cubed
4 tomatoes, diced

Mix the ingredients together and toss with your favourite dressing. Serve immediately.

Spring Gardens Salad (neutral)

Another simple biogenic salad, this dish goes particularly well with Racy Red Cheese dressing, Light Vinaigrette or Avocado Delight.

2 C radicchio, torn into small pieces
1 C alfalfa sprouts
1 punnet of mustard and cress
1 C thinly sliced cos lettuce
2 small carrots, washed but not peeled, sliced thinly
1 turnip, sliced thinly into matchsticks
24 black olives, stoned
4 tomatoes, sectioned into quarters
chives or *herbs (optional)*

Put all the ingredients (except the tomatoes) into a large bowl and toss with a salad dressing of your choice. Place the tomato quarters around the side and sprinkle with some chopped chives or fresh herbs if you like.

Branton's Booster (protein)

This protein-based biogenic salad is particularly good when you feel the need for something quite substantial, especially if you are doing a lot of exercise. As it contains sprouted sunflower seeds, this is a salad that really feels as if it sticks to your ribs.

1 C sprouted sunflower seeds
2 C chopped chicory
2 C alfalfa sprouts
1 C lentil sprouts or *mung-bean sprouts*
5 tomatoes, sliced thinly
3 celery stalks, cut lengthways three or four times, then chopped crossways finely
2 green peppers, seeded and chopped
1½ C chopped fennel

Toss all the ingredients together and serve with Horsey Tomato Dressing or Light Vinaigrette.

Cress Special (neutral)

This is an ultra-light salad which contains no oil. The combination of lemon and tamari is quite delightful.

1 C curled cress, watercress or *roquette*
1 C alfalfa sprouts

^{1}/2 C lentil sprouts
2 sticks of celery, cut lengthways three or four times then chopped crossways
    finely
1 avocado, peeled and cubed
3 tbsp tamari
1 clove of garlic, finely chopped
2 tbsp parsley or fresh basil, finely chopped
juice of 2 lemons

Toss the ingredients into a bowl, sprinkle with the lemon juice and
tamari and serve.

The Green Light (neutral)

I like to serve this salad with Creamy Lemon Dressing.

^{1}/2 C alfalfa sprouts
^{1}/2 C mung-bean sprouts
^{1}/2 C fenugreek sprouts
^{1}/2 C sunflower-seed sprouts
^{1}/2 C chicory, sliced finely
^{1}/2 C cos lettuce
4 spring onions, chopped finely
4 tomatoes, chopped
1 courgette, sliced finely
2 stalks of celery, cut lengthways three or four times then chopped
    crossways finely
1 large beetroot, grated finely
2 large carrots, grated finely

Mix all the ingredients (except the grated carrots and beetroot) in a
bowl and toss with salad dressing. Arrange the carrots and the
beetroot separately around the rim to decorate. Serve immediately.

Crudités

One of my favourite hors d'oeuvres or salads is a platter of crudités
– crunchy raw vegetables and fruit sliced or chopped so that you can
pick the pieces up with your fingers. They can be eaten dipped into
sauce (see Chapter 26) or simply sprinkled with a light dressing and
a few toasted fennel or caraway seeds. The important thing is how
you prepare them.

Sticks and Matchsticks

Make sticks from carrots, turnips, courgettes, cucumbers, celery and pineapple. To make matchsticks, just keep chopping until you get 'baby sticks' that are about the size of a match (you can also make matchsticks from green and red peppers). To keep sticks fresh, put them into a bowl of cold water with a squeeze of lemon and refrigerate them.

Slices

Some vegetables are particularly nice sliced diagonally. This makes larger pieces for better 'dunkers'. Try diagonal slices of cucumber, carrot and white radish. Very thin slices of small beetroot, Jerusalem artichoke, kohlrabi and turnip are also nice. Large apples sliced crossways can be used as 'bread' for open-air sandwiches. Sweet peppers cut crossways make attractive rings. Try cutting ½in slices of peppers and placing around a bundle of carrot or celery sticks.

Whole Vegetables

Button mushrooms with their stalks on, whole baby carrots, the small centre stalks from a head of celery, whole young green beans that have been topped and tailed, florets of cauliflower, radishes, young spring onions – simply trimmed and rinsed, they all make great crudités.

Wedges

Wedges of tomato, chicory, iceberg lettuce, oranges, tangerines, apples and pears.

It is nice to garnish a plate of crudités with some half-slices of lemon, sprigs of watercress, parsley or mint and some of your favourite sprouts.

Bioactive Salads

Greek Delight Plus (protein)

A new twist on a classic Greek salad, with extra protein added in the form of feta cheese.

4in piece of cucumber
4–8 oz feta cheese

8 oz tomatoes
1 dozen black olives
3 C fresh alfalfa sprouts

For the Dressing
1 clove of garlic, chopped finely
3 tbsp chopped fresh basil
1 tbsp lemon juice
1 tbsp virgin olive oil
black pepper

Chop the cucumber, feta cheese and tomatoes into small pieces. Mix them in a bowl together with the black olives. Mix the dressing ingredients together in a screw-top jar by shaking them. Pour the dressing over the salad and toss. Then arrange on a bed of alfalfa sprouts and serve on a platter.

Spinach Splendour (protein)

This delicious complete-meal salad is set off by a subtle dressing based on dry white wine and walnut oil.

3 oz spinach leaves
1½ C alfalfa sprouts
6 to 8 radishes, sliced finely
4 oz mushrooms, sliced finely
4 hard-boiled eggs, either chopped finely or grated

For the Dressing
2 tbsp walnut oil
3 tbsp lemon juice
½ lemon rind grated
1 tbsp freshly grated root ginger
2 tbsp dry white wine
2 cloves of garlic, chopped finely
1 tsp vegetable bouillon powder or *sea-salt* or *soy sauce*
black pepper

Wash the spinach leaves and dry them thoroughly in a spinner or in a towel. Combine all the ingredients of the salad together in a large bowl. Mix the ingredients of the dressing together by shaking well in a screw-top jar. Pour dressing over the salad and toss. Add the grated or chopped hard-boiled eggs on the top and serve chilled.

Scottish Pine (protein)

The combination of lamb's lettuce with pine kernels is unbeatable – another top favourite.

8 oz tomatoes, diced
6 radishes, sliced finely
6 spring onions, chopped finely
8 oz lamb's lettuce
3 tbsp parsley, chopped finely
1 C alfalfa or fenugreek sprouts
3 oz pine kernels

For the Dressing
1 tbsp cider vinegar
3 tbsp sunflower oil
1 clove of garlic, chopped finely
1 tsp vegetable bouillon powder or sea-salt
1 tsp Meaux mustard
black pepper

Combine the finely chopped ingredients with the lamb's lettuce and the sprouts. Mix the dressing ingredients together in a screw-top bottle and shake well. Pour the dressing over the salad, toss, and garnish with the pine kernels. Serve chilled.

Celeriac Special (protein)

We've grown celeriac in our garden all winter. It is a pleasure to have this crunchy, delicately flavoured organic root as part of almost any salad.

4 medium celeriac, grated finely
2 medium carrots, scrubbed but not peeled, grated finely
4 oz chopped pecans
10 chives, leaves chopped very finely
1/2 red pepper, seeded and chopped finely
1/2 green pepper, seeded and chopped finely
mayonnaise for dressing (see pages 204–7)

12 black olives, stones removed
outer leaves from a head of radicchio or chicory

Mix all the ingredients except the olives and the leaves together, dressed with a good mayonnaise. Arrange on a bed of chicory or radicchio leaves, decorate with the olives, and serve immediately.

Raita (protein)

A delicious cucumber salad which can be made with either a low-fat dairy yogurt or a savoury nut or seed cream.

3 finely diced carrots
handful of fresh peas
1 large cucumber, sliced lengthways, then crossways, in order to produce
   slivers each about 1½-2in long
1 C low-fat yogurt or seed cream or nut cream
juice of 1 lemon
2 tbsp fresh mint leaves, finely chopped
crisp salad greens

Make sure the carrots, peas and cucumber are chilled thoroughly. Take a little yogurt or seed or nut cream to which you have added the finely chopped fresh mint leaves and the lemon juice and pour over the salad, mixing well. Serve on crisp salad greens.

Devil's Delight (neutral)

Raw beetroot has remarkable properties for detoxification; it's also an excellent source of vitamin C and a number of important minerals. And it is delicious – particularly married with fresh apples. Once you taste it you will wonder how you could ever eat this beautiful red root vegetable cooked.

3 raw beetroot
3 green apples
3 white radishes

For the Dressing
2 tbsp sunflower oil
1 tbsp lemon juice
1 tsp Meaux mustard

3 tbsp chopped parsley
4 spring onions, chopped
finely ground black pepper
1 tsp vegetable bouillon powder

Grate the beetroot, apples and radishes, preferably in a food processor, then mix together in a bowl. Put the dressing ingredients in a screw-top jar and shake. Pour your dressing over the salad and toss.

Green Glory Salad (neutral)

This is a delightful, crunchy summer salad which goes equally well garnished with chopped eggs as a protein meal or served with a baked potato or a starchy soup as a starch meal.

8 oz Chinese leaves, shredded finely
1 green pepper (seeds removed), chopped
3 tbsp lovage leaves, chopped finely or fresh mint, chopped finely
4 sticks of celery, cut lengthways three or four times, then chopped crossways finely
3 spring onions, sliced diagonally

For the Dressing
4 tbsp mayonnaise
2 tbsp orange juice
grated rind from 1/2 orange
2 tbsp chopped parsley
1 tsp vegetable bouillon powder or sea-salt
2 cloves of garlic, chopped finely

Shred, chop and prepare the vegetables and put them into a large bowl. Mix dressing ingredients in a screw-top jar and shake well. Pour the dressing over the salad and toss. Garnish with lovage leaves or fresh mint. Serve chilled.

Tomato Treasures (neutral)

This stuffed tomato salad is delicious and so pretty to serve.

8 tomatoes
1 avocado, peeled and stoned

juice of 2 lemons
2 cloves of garlic, crushed
3 tbsp finely chopped basil
dash of Tabasco sauce to taste
1 tsp vegetable bouillon powder or *sea-salt*
2 C fresh alfalfa sprouts
2 oz lamb's lettuce
6 spring onions, chopped diagonally

For the Dressing
1 tbsp olive oil
1 tbsp lemon juice
3 tbsp chopped fresh parsley
1 tsp vegetable bouillon powder
1 clove of garlic, chopped finely
1 tbsp chopped fresh basil
black pepper (optional)

Slice the lid from each tomato and remove the insides with a spoon. Mix the insides in a blender or food processor with all the other ingredients except the alfalfa sprouts, the lamb's lettuce and the spring onions; then spoon back into the tomato shells. Toss the salad made out of the alfalfa sprouts, lamb's lettuce and spring onions with the dressing and season with black pepper if desired. Spread onto a platter and place the tomatoes on top. Serve chilled.

Jerusalem Artichoke Salad (neutral)

A sweet and crunchy winter salad, this dish is another favourite. It is simple to prepare but tastes like something very special.

6 Jerusalem artichokes, grated finely
3 carrots, grated finely
1 apple, chopped finely
3 tbsp parsley, chopped finely
3 stalks of celery, cut lengthways two or three times, then chopped crossways finely
3/4 C Chinese leaves, chopped finely

For the Dressing
mayonnaise (see pages 204–7)
cayenne pepper
garlic

Mix together and serve with the dressing. You can turn this salad into an excellent protein salad by serving it with a seed cheese or by sprinkling some pumpkin or sunflower seeds over the top.

Watercress Salad (neutral)
This is a special treat for me because I love the slightly bitter taste and the beautiful dark green colour of fresh watercress.

3 C cos lettuce, torn into small pieces
1 bunch of watercress, cut into ¹/₂in lengths
4 spring onions, chopped finely
³/₄ C courgettes, grated
2 carrots, grated
4 tomatoes, quartered
3–4 tbsp sunflower seeds (optional)

Combine all the ingredients and serve with a vinaigrette (see page 208). This salad can be turned into a beautiful protein dish by sprinkling 3–4 tbsp of sunflower seeds on the top.

Root-is-Best Salad (neutral)
This salad is a pleasurable statement of how delicious the humble root vegetable can be.

2 turnips, grated finely
3 fresh parsnips, scrubbed but not peeled, and grated
2 carrots, scrubbed but not peeled, and grated
1 sweet potato, peeled and grated or 1 potato, grated
3 spring onions, chopped finely
¹/₂ red pepper, deseeded and chopped finely
¹/₂ green pepper, deseeded and chopped finely
1 tbsp chopped summer savory or lovage
juice of 1 lemon

2 C Chinese leaves, or *lettuce, finely grated or chopped*
mayonnaise (see pages 204–7)
spring or filtered water

Mix all vegetable ingredients together except the Chinese leaves
and pour lemon juice over them. Toss well and serve on a bed of
finely grated Chinese leaves or lettuce with a good mayonnaise
which has been thinned with a little spring or filtered water.

Bulgar Salad with Endive (starch)

A delicious and substantial dish which, thanks to the endive and the
bulgar wheat, is high in vitamin E. The contrast between the rich
graininess of the bulgar wheat and the delicate flavour of the endive
is most pleasing.

4 oz bulgar wheat
1 endive
6 spring onions
a punnet of salad cress

For the Dressing
1 tbsp sunflower oil
3 tsp chopped fresh parsley
juice of ½ lemon
rind of ½ lemon
1 tsp white-wine vinegar
1 tsp vegetable bouillon powder or *sea-salt*
black pepper
1 clove of garlic, chopped finely

Soak the bulgar wheat overnight or for at least three hours in
enough water to cover. Then drain excess water. Put dressing
ingredients in a screw-top jar and mix by shaking well. Add endive,
onions and salad cress to the bulgar wheat in a bowl and mix. Pour
the dressing over the salad and toss.

Celebration Salad (starch)

This main-dish salad is another beautiful marriage between
vegetable and grain, set off by the delicate flavour of sesame oil,
lemon and orange which go into the dressing.

6 oz long-grain brown rice
3 large carrots, sliced in very thin discs
1 C fenugreek sprouts
1/4 cucumber, sliced finely
4 oz garden peas
black pepper
1/4 tsp vegetable bouillon powder
a few sprigs of mint or lovage

For the Dressing
juice of 1/2 lemon
juice of 1/2 orange
2 tsp sesame oil
1/2 tsp grated or ground nutmeg
2 tbsp finely chopped fresh mint

Put the rice into a saucepan. Cover with about 2in of water, bring to the boil and simmer for 35 minutes or until tender. Put the dressing ingredients together and shake in a screw-top jar. Pour over the rice whilst it is still warm and combine carefully. Let the mixture cool completely. Add the vegetables to the rice. Season with a little black pepper and vegetable bouillon powder, garnish with mint or lovage.

Potato Supreme (starch)

This is a light and delicately flavoured potato salad, very different from the stodgy, oily variety which most people know.

1 lb potatoes, preferably organic
1/2 cucumber, diced
5 sticks of celery, diced
2 large carrots, diced
3 spring onions, diced
3 tbsp finely chopped fresh parsley
2 cloves of garlic, chopped finely
1 tsp dill, chopped finely

For the Dressing
5 tbsp mayonnaise (see pages 204–7)
2 tbsp lemon juice
1 tsp Meaux mustard

1 tsp vegetable bouillon powder or *soy sauce*
black pepper

Scrub the potatoes carefully but do not peel. Add them to a saucepan of boiling water and simmer for 15 to 20 minutes until they are tender. Drain and cool, then dice. Mix the ingredients of the dressing together with a spoon and add to the potatoes. Now chill and when completely chilled add the remaining ingredients and serve.

26
Dips and Dressings

THE FRESH VEGETABLES, herbs and other delicacies that you put into a salad are only half the story: the other half is the dressing. So splendid are some of the dressings that you can use on the biogenic diet that they will undoubtedly delight your family and friends while at the same time helping you trim away the excess fat.

Dressings come in two varieties: they can be protein in nature, like some of the lovely seed dressings and sunflower creams, or they can be neutral (and used on either protein or starch salads) as is the usual Italian or French dressing to which most people are accustomed.

So filling are some of the protein dressings that they are all the extra protein for a meal which you will need when served with a large, delicious biogenic salad. Many recipes can be for either a dip or a dressing, depending upon how thick you make them. The dips are best used for crudités; the dressings are best poured over salads which have been grated or chopped or over sprouts.

Mayonnaise (protein)

This is a classic mayonnaise which can be varied by adding different herbs, Dijon mustard, curry powder or garlic to it, depending upon the use to which you want to put it.

2 raw egg yolks at room temperature
1 tsp dry mustard
dash of cayenne
1 tsp vegetable bouillon powder
juice of 1 lemon

*2 C salad oil (this can be a mixture of olive oil with sesame or sunflower oil
   or, for a light dressing, it can be entirely sunflower or corn oil)*

In a food processor or blender, thoroughly blend the egg yolks with
the mustard, the cayenne and the vegetable bouillon powder. Add 2
tbsp of lemon juice. While still blending add the oil, a few drops at a
time, very slowly until about half the oil has been blended. Finally
beat in the remaining oil, about two tablespoons at a time. This
dressing will keep in the refrigerator for 5 to 6 days.

Sunny Tomato Special (protein)

A surprising combination of the tangy flavour of tomatoes with the
richness of fresh sunflower seeds.

6 tomatoes or *1 medium tin of tomatoes*
1 C sunflower seeds
1 tsp vegetable bouillon powder or *soy sauce*
1 clove of garlic, finely chopped
juice of 2 lemons
1 tbsp fresh finely chopped parsley or *fresh basil (if you can't get the fresh
   herbs you may use much smaller quantities of the dried ones)*

Put the ingredients together in a blender or food processor and
blend thoroughly. If you want a thicker consistency add more
sunflower seeds (but remember the dressing will thicken as it
stands); if you want a thinner consistency add a little water. Chill
thoroughly before use. Made with fresh tomatoes this dressing will
keep for two days in the refrigerator; made with tinned tomatoes it
will keep for four or five.

Nut Mayonnaise (protein)

A delicious alternative mayonnaise which goes beautifully with
crudités and also as a garnish for lightly steamed vegetables.

4 oz cashews
1 C spring water
2 cloves of garlic, finely chopped
juice of 1 lemon
1 tsp vegetable bouillon powder or *sea-salt* or *soy sauce*
spring onions, finely chopped

Blend together well in a food processor or blender, chill and serve. This recipe will keep for four or five days covered in the refrigerator.

Soya Cottage Cheese (protein)

Light, high in protein, low in fat and simply yummy.

2 C soybean curd (see Resources for stockists)
¾ C nut mayonnaise or *tahini mayonnaise* or *plain mayonnaise*
1 tsp vegetable bouillon powder or *soy sauce* or *sea-salt*
1 tsp caraway seeds
1 tsp mild curry powder
1 clove of garlic, chopped finely
handful of fresh herbs (mint, lovage, lemon balm) if available
2 tbsp chopped chives

Mash the soybean curd well with a fork, add the other ingredients and blend. Chill before serving. This dressing will keep up to a week in the refrigerator.

Raw Houmus (protein)

2 C sprouted chickpeas (sprouted for two to three days)
1 clove of garlic, chopped finely
3 tbsp tahini
juice of 3 lemons
enough water to thin
1 tsp vegetable bouillon powder or *2 tsp soy sauce*
3 tsp chopped spring onions or *chives*

Put the ingredients (except the chives or spring onions) into a food processor or blender and blend thoroughly. Then mix in the chopped chives or spring onions and chill. This dressing will keep for two to three days in the refrigerator.

Extralite Tahini Mayonnaise (protein)

This mayonnaise makes a delicious dip for crudités. Warning: it's *very* rich.

1 C tahini
1 C water
1 clove of garlic, finely chopped
2 tbsp chopped fresh parsley
1 tsp vegetable bouillon powder
juice of 3 lemons

Put the ingredients into a blender or food processor or mix them together by hand until you get a smooth consistency. Refrigerate. This dressing will keep up to a week in the refrigerator.

Tahini Mayonnaise (protein)

This mayonnaise is also delicious as a dip for crudités or served over steamed vegetables.

juice of 2 lemons or ¼ C cider vinegar
½ tsp vegetable bouillon powder or soy sauce
4 tbsp tahini
½ C water
1 clove of chopped garlic
¼ C olive oil

Mix all the ingredients except the olive oil in a blender or food processor until thoroughly blended. Add the olive oil very slowly, as much as you need to thicken. Store in a glass jar in the refrigerator. Will keep for four to five days.

Sprout Splendour (protein)

1 C alfalfa sprouts
4 sprigs of celery, chopped very finely
1 tsp vegetable bouillon powder or 2 tbsp tamari
¾ C sunflower oil
juice of 2 lemons
1 tbsp finely chopped onion
1 tbsp sesame seeds
1 tsp Dijon mustard

Blend thoroughly and serve on a fresh green salad or use as a dip. Must be eaten same day – does not keep well.

Light Vinaigrette (neutral)

2 tbsp cider vinegar
4 tbsp sesame oil
1/2 tsp Meaux mustard
1/2 tsp tarragon
1/2 tsp chervil
1/2 tsp vegetable bouillon powder or *sea-salt*

Mix the vinegar, oil, mustard, herbs and bouillon powder or salt together and blend well by putting them all into a jar with a screw-top lid and shaking thoroughly.

Celery Special (neutral)

This is a surprisingly fresh and unusually flavoured dressing which goes well with an all-green salad. I particularly like it with lamb's lettuce.

1/2 C olive oil
1/4 C celery seeds
3 spring onions, chopped finely
1 clove of garlic, chopped finely
1/2 tsp marjoram
2 tsp fresh parsley, chopped finely
1 tsp vegetable bouillon powder or *a little sea-salt*

Blend well by shaking in a screw-top jar.

Horsey Tomato Dressing (neutral)

This is a delightful dressing to serve over finely sliced cucumbers in summertime.

1/2 C olive oil
juice from 2 lemons
1/2 tsp Dijon mustard
2 tsp horseradish
1 clove of garlic, crushed
2 fresh tomatoes

¹/₂ tsp sesame seeds
1 tsp vegetable bouillon powder or other seasoning

Blend well in a blender or food processor and serve chilled.

Parsley Cream (protein)

This is a low-fat salad dressing based on yogurt. It's particularly good served on biogenic salads of sprouts, cucumbers and tomatoes. It also makes a nice addition to a slaw.

1 C natural low-fat yogurt
juice of 1 lemon
¹/₂ tsp dill
small onion, chopped
2 tsp chopped parsley
¹/₂ tsp vegetable bouillon powder or soy sauce

Blend well together by hand or in a blender. Will keep four to five days in a refrigerator.

Pink Yogurt Dressing (protein)

Not as good as pink champagne, perhaps, but sheer delight on sprouts and cucumber.

1 C thick yogurt
4 tbsp tomato purée
1 tsp Meaux mustard
¹/₂ clove garlic, chopped finely
¹/₂ tsp vegetable bouillon powder
1 tbsp chopped shallots or spring onions

Mix everything but the shallots together well – in a blender if possible. Then add the shallots and finish mixing. Serve chilled. Will keep up to five days in the refrigerator.

Green Dream (protein)

This dressing is ideal for a potato salad. It's also delicious on finely sliced tomatoes.

2 cucumbers
3 spring onions, chopped finely
juice of 1 lemon
1 tsp horseradish
1/2 tsp vegetable bouillon powder or soy sauce or sea-salt
1 C natural yogurt, seed cheese or home-made mayonnaise

Blend together in a food processor all the ingredients except the mayonnaise, seed cheese or yogurt. Fold into the mayonnaise, seed cheese or yogurt and chill. Will not keep for more than a day.

Avocado Delight (neutral)

This is a superb dip or dressing, and very rich indeed. Excellent on a sprout salad or as a dip for crudités.

1 avocado, peeled and stoned
juice of 1 lemon
juice of 1/2 orange
1 small onion, chopped finely
1 clove of garlic, chopped finely
handful of fresh herbs – mint, parsley or basil
black pepper

Blend all the ingredients in a food processor or blender and serve. This dip will not keep for more than one day in a refrigerator.

Creamy Lemon Dressing (protein)

juice of 2 lemons
2 tbsp chopped cashews
1/2 tsp vegetable bouillon powder
1/2 C sunflower oil

Combine the ingredients (except the oil) together in a blender or food processor and blend thoroughly. Then add the oil slowly, drop by drop.

French Spice (neutral)

A pleasant light dressing that seems to complement any salad.

juice of 2 lemons

2 ripe tomatoes
1 clove of garlic
12 chives, chopped finely
1 tsp powdered kelp (optional)
1/3 C sunflower oil
1 tsp cayenne
1 tbsp tamari
1 tbsp Dijon mustard
1 tsp vegetable bouillon powder

Blend the ingredients together in a food processor or blender until thoroughly mixed. This dressing may be refrigerated and kept for up to four days.

Italian Dressing (neutral)

Another classic dressing. I like this one on biogenic salads. It also goes well with my favourite greens such as lamb's lettuce, roquette, American land cress and curly cress served on their own and sprinkled with parsley.

1 pint virgin olive oil
2 tbsp paprika
2 tbsp finely chopped fresh basil
2 tsp vegetable bouillon powder or *2 tbsp tahini*
1/2 tsp dried oregano
pinch of cayenne
pinch of kelp (optional)
1/4 C chopped fennel
1/2 tsp finely chopped red pepper

Put the ingredients into a screw-top jar and shake vigorously until well mixed. You may thin this dressing with water if it seems too thick. It will keep well for up to 10 days in the refrigerator.

Wild Carrot Dressing (protein)

This dressing is one of my favourites. It goes well either on a salad or on steamed vegetables.

3 large carrots, washed and cut into small pieces
10 chives, chopped finely

1 tsp vegetable bouillon powder
1 C blanched almonds (preferably soaked overnight in 1–2 C spring or filtered water)
2 tsp chopped parsley

Put all the ingredients into a food processor or blender and blend with as much water as you need to make the dressing the consistency you want. It's best to leave it thick if you want to use it as a dip, or make it thinner as a dressing to pour over salads.

Green Glory Dressing (protein)

This dressing is an absolute cinch to make if you have fresh herbs in the garden; you may be amazed to find how many herbs and of what different varieties you can use to make it.

2 tbsp virgin olive oil
2 tbsp lemon juice
¾ C fresh natural yogurt or ⅓ C cashews mixed with ½ C water to make a cashew cream
2–8 tbsp fresh herbs from the garden (whatever you have available: lovage, mint, apple mint, lemon mint, balm, chives, spring onions, etc.)

Place all the ingredients in a blender or food processor and blend thoroughly until the dressing turns green. This dressing will keep for four to five days in the refrigerator.

Racy Red Cheese (protein)

This delicious dip or dressing can be served with crudités, over a salad or added to freshly steamed or wok-fried vegetables. It's a beautiful pink colour and has a refreshing zippy taste.

1 C cashews or pine nuts
1 C filtered or spring water
1 tsp vegetable bouillon powder or sea-salt
½ tsp caraway seeds
juice of 2 lemons
½ C pimentos
4 chopped spring onions or chives

Mix all the ingredients (except the chives or spring onions) in a blender or food processor until smooth. Blend in the chives or spring onions by hand and serve. This dip may be kept in the refrigerator for four to five days.

27
Seductive Soups

THERE WAS A time when a good soup formed the basis of a main meal for the whole family – and in many parts of the world it still does. I often use the heartier full-bodied soups in this way – particularly in winter. I take whatever vegetables I can find in the garden or in the refrigerator, chop them and put them into a big pot with fresh or dried herbs and perhaps a cereal such as millet, barley, rice or buckwheat. The results are wonderful – particularly if you use vegetable bouillon as your stock. Once you get the hang of it you simply can't help but make a good soup.

The soups in this section fall into two categories – those which are biogenic and bioactive and therefore either served cold or heated to no more than about 110°F (43°C) in order to preserve the enzymes they contain, and the traditional old-fashioned soups which most of our ancestors lived on. Try both types – as main dishes and as side-dishes to go with total-meal salads. I hope you'll like them as much as I and my family do.

Biogenic Soup (protein)

This protein soup, which is made from biogenic and bioactive foods (in effect by turning a biogenic salad into a soup) is not only light and delicious, it also offers a full complement of high-quality protein plus a very high level of vitamins and minerals.

sprouted seeds or grain (alfalfa, lentils, mung beans, fenugreek, etc.)
seed cheese (any variety) or *yogurt*
2 tsp vegetable bouillon powder
spring or *filtered water as needed*

Optional

sunflower seeds
selection of fresh or *dried herbs*
avocado
carrots, tomatoes, mushrooms, parsley, garlic, etc.

Put two or three handfuls of mixed sprouted beans or grains in a blender or food processor. Cover with 1½ C of thin seed cheese or yogurt and blend. Add the seasoning and extra ingredients (perhaps a finely chopped clove of garlic, 2 tbsp of chopped parsley, ½ avocado or some mushrooms). Add to this the vegetable bouillon powder and blend well, adding spring or filtered water to this as needed. Can be served either cold or heated to just above body temperature. Caution: do not overheat or you destroy enzymes present in these living foods.

Leek and Potato Soup (starch)

This is a delicious and creamy soup which goes beautifully with a neutral biogenic or bioactive salad to make up a whole meal. It is a starch soup.

1 large onion, sliced
3 medium-sized leeks, sliced lengthwise, washed and chopped into fine pieces
3 large potatoes, peeled and sliced
1 tbsp olive oil
¾ pint spring or *filtered water (more if needed)*
2 tsp vegetable bouillon powder
½ tsp freshly grated nutmeg or *ground black pepper*

Brown the onion, leeks and potatoes in the olive oil for ten minutes until onion becomes translucent. Boil the water in a kettle and pour over the browned vegetables. Bring to the boil, add the vegetable bouillon powder, and simmer for 10–15 minutes. Liquidize in a food processor or blender and serve hot with grated nutmeg (or ground pepper if preferred) sprinkled on top of each bowl.

Barley Mushroom Soup (starch)

A starch soup, this is a beautiful winter meal which is welcoming, warming and friendly. The ideal thing for a cosy winter evening in front of the fire.

½ C barley
2 pints spring or filtered water
3 tbsp olive oil
3 cloves of garlic, minced
2 large onions, chopped finely
1 lb fresh mushrooms, sliced thinly
3 tsp vegetable bouillon powder
1 avocado
½ C dry white wine
freshly ground black pepper

Cook the barley in half of the water until tender, then add the remaining water. In another pan sauté the garlic and the onions in the olive oil; when they are softened, add the mushrooms. When everything is tender add to the barley and cook for another 35 minutes. Add the bouillon powder. Mash the avocado with a fork or blend in a blender or food processor and stir into the soup with the dry white wine just before serving. Add a generous grinding of black pepper.

Curried Pumpkin Soup (starch)

This starch soup is charming and spicy and goes beautifully with a sprout salad.

2 medium onions, chopped finely
1 clove of garlic, chopped finely
2 C fresh pumpkin, cut into small cubes (substitute marrow for this if you wish)
½ lb mushrooms, sliced
2 tbsp olive oil
3 C boiled water or stock
½ tsp ground cumin
½ tsp coriander
½ tsp cinnamon
½ tsp ground ginger
½ tsp dry mustard

2 tsp vegetable bouillon powder or *sea-salt*
pinch of cayenne
juice of 2 fresh lemons

Sauté the onions, the garlic, the pumpkin and the mushrooms gently in olive oil until soft. Add the boiled water and cook for ten minutes. Add seasonings and cook for another five or ten minutes. Place in a blender or food processor and blend thoroughly. Add freshly squeezed lemon juice and serve.

Bioactive Avocado and Tomato Soup (neutral)
This neutral soup is light and spicy. You can serve it hot or cold.

8 ripe tomatoes
1 ripe avocado
2 spring onions, chopped finely
¹/₄ tsp ground dill seed
pinch of cayenne
1 C spring or *filtered water*
2 tsp vegetable bouillon powder
1 tsp kelp (optional)
1 green pepper, chopped finely

Blend all the ingredients (except the finely chopped green pepper and two of the tomatoes) in a blender or food processor. Heat gently to warm but not above 115°F (46°C). Chop the last two tomatoes and add with the green pepper when you serve.

Chilled Cucumber Soup (protein)
This delightful protein soup 'can't be beat' on a hot summer day.

1 large cucumber
2 C natural yogurt or *seed milk*
4 tbsp finely chopped mint
2 tsp vegetable bouillon powder
¹/₄ tsp crushed poppy seed (optional)
ice (optional)

Chop cucumber and blend in blender or food processor with chilled yogurt or seed milk. You may add a few cubes of ice to make it colder if you wish. After blending for two minutes, add the vegetable bouillon powder and continue to blend with the ice. Finally add the chopped mint and blend again very briefly. Pour into bowls and serve immediately with a little chopped mint or crushed poppy seed sprinkled on top.

Gazpacho (neutral)

Another delicious cold neutral summer soup which you can make as spicy as you like.

6 ripe tomatoes, chopped
1/2 cucumber, chopped
juice of 1 lemon
2 tsp vegetable bouillon powder
1 tsp kelp (optional)
1 clove garlic, finely chopped
1/2 red pepper, finely chopped
1/2 green pepper, finely chopped
4 spring onions, finely chopped
3 tbsp parsley, finely chopped
cayenne pepper to taste

Keeping aside a small portion of the tomatoes and of the chopped cucumber, put the rest of the tomatoes and cucumber, the lemon juice, bouillon powder, kelp (if desired) and garlic in a food processor or blender and liquidize. Add the peppers, spring onions and parsley and mix well, season to taste with cayenne pepper and serve with the tomatoes and cucumber you have kept aside.

Corn Soup (starch)

A bioactive starch dish, this soup is uncooked and can either be served cold or warm.

2 fresh ears of corn
1/2 pint warm spring or filtered water
2 spring onions, chopped
1 tbsp olive oil
1 tsp vegetable bouillon powder
1 tbsp tahini (optional)

¼ red pepper, chopped
¼ green pepper, chopped
1 tbsp watercress, chopped finely

Wash the corn and cut the kernels off the cob with a knife. Mix together with the water, spring onions, olive oil and vegetable bouillon powder, season with tahini (if desired), and blend until creamy in a blender or food processor. Add the chopped peppers and watercress to each portion.

Bioactive Asparagus Soup (protein)
A very special uncooked but heated protein soup, this dish is a delicate marriage of the unusual taste and aroma of the asparagus with the rich sensuous quality of the cashews.

¾ C cashew nuts
3 C spring or filtered water
1 bunch fresh raw asparagus (tips only)
3 sticks celery
2 tsp vegetable bouillon powder
2 tbsp fresh lovage, chopped finely (optional)
2 tbsp chopped parsley

Place the cashew nuts in a food processor with 1 C hot water and blend thoroughly until reduced to a cream. Add to the mixture the other ingredients, keeping aside the chopped parsley. Heat thoroughly but do not boil. Serve with a sprinkling of parsley.

Scottish Barley Soup (starch)
Another starch dish, this is one of my favourite hearty soups. I like it best on chilly autumn evenings. It goes beautifully well with a mixed green salad full of fresh herbs.

1 C barley
1 litre spring or filtered water
2 onions chopped
3 carrots, chopped into cubes
6 sticks of celery, diced
4 oz mushrooms, chopped (optional)
1 tbsp olive oil

1 tin tomatoes or *6 fresh tomatoes*
3 cloves of garlic, chopped finely
2 tbsp parsley, chopped finely

Cook the barley for an hour in the water. In a separate pan fry the onions, carrots, celery and (if you like) mushrooms in the olive oil. Add to the barley along with the tomatoes and garlic and simmer for 20 minutes. Serve piping hot, sprinkled with fresh parsley. If you prefer a smooth soup, liquidize it in a blender or food processor.

Seductive Celery Cream (protein)

I find this protein soup utterly irresistible, but then I have a special passion for cashews, whose creamy qualities help them marry well with crunchy celery.

1 litre spring or *filtered water*
1/2 C celery leaves and tops, chopped
3/4 C cashews
1 medium onion, chopped finely
2 C chopped celery bottoms
2 medium carrots, diced
1 C fresh or *frozen peas (optional)*
1 tbsp olive oil
3 tsp vegetable bouillon powder or *other seasoning*

Put into a blender half the water, celery tops and leaves and cashews and blend thoroughly. Meanwhile sauté the onion, celery bottoms, carrots and peas in the olive oil. Then add everything together with the vegetable bouillon powder, bring to the boil with the remainder of the water, and simmer for no more than 10 minutes. Serve warm.

High Potassium Broth (starch)

This is an excellent dish to use not only as a soup but also as a broth to drink if you wish to miss a meal or even a whole day's meals, or just as a substitute for tea or coffee during the day. To use the soup as a broth you discard the vegetables. As a soup you drink it vegetables and all. This broth makes an excellent bouillon to use in other soups.

4 medium potatoes (including skins), diced
4 finely diced carrots
3 finely diced celery sticks
2 C green peas
1 large onion, chopped
2 cloves garlic, crushed
discarded leaves from lettuce, cabbage, cauliflower, Brussels sprouts, etc.
1 tbsp vegetable bouillon powder
2 litres spring or filtered water
3 tbsp fresh parsley, finely chopped

Clean and chop the leaves and vegetables, discarding any wilted parts, and put into the pot with all the other ingredients. Bring to a boil and let simmer for two hours, then strain. Garnish with chopped parsley and serve.

Garlic Soup (starch)

This starch soup is for garlic lovers only. My daughter Susannah and I constantly fight over how much garlic should go into soups, salads, sauces and other dishes. I am an enormous garlic fan; Susannah believes that one whiff of garlic is enough to keep her intoxicated for a week. This soup is definitely of my own devising: it is also absolutely delicious. Susannah, alas, has never tasted it. The mere sight of the recipe would make her cringe.

3 potatoes (with skins on)
2 carrots
3 sticks of celery
1 large onion
1 litre spring or filtered water
2 large heads garlic
pinch of oregano
1/2 tsp thyme
pinch of sage
dash of cayenne
2 tbsp fresh parsley, finely chopped
1 tbsp vegetable bouillon powder

Cut potatoes, carrots, celery and onion into cubes and add to water that has been brought to the boil. Break garlic into individual cloves and add these together with the herbs and spices. Add bouillon powder and bring to the boil; simmer for 20 to 30 minutes. Put soup into a blender or food processor and blend, or strain vegetables from it and serve as a clear broth with parsley sprinkled on top.

Courgette Tomato Soup (neutral)

This neutral soup is beautifully light with a delicate Italian flavour to it.

3 medium courgettes, diced
3 sticks of celery, chopped finely
4 spring onions, chopped
1 large carrot, diced
1 clove of garlic, crushed or chopped
1 tbsp olive oil
6 tomatoes, peeled and chopped
1 tbsp fresh basil, chopped finely or ½ tsp oregano
3 tsp vegetable bouillon powder or other seasoning

Sauté all the vegetables (except the tomatoes) and garlic in the olive oil for five minutes. Then add the tomatoes and pour in enough boiling water to cover. Bring to the boil and simmer for 20–30 minutes. Serve sprinkled with fresh basil or oregano and season according to taste.

Split-Pea Soup (starch)

Another hearty starch soup which goes well with a biogenic or green salad.

1 C dried split peas which have been soaked in water to cover overnight
1 large onion, chopped
2 medium carrots, diced
2 sticks of celery, diced
1 litre spring or filtered water
1 tbsp vegetable bouillon powder
2 tbsp chopped fresh herbs as available (parsley, lovage, sage, pot marjoram)

After the peas have been washed and soaked overnight, put them in a pot with all the vegetables and cover with water. Bring to the boil and simmer for 1½ hours until the peas are tender. Add the vegetable bouillon powder and fresh herbs five minutes before serving. If you want a smooth soup, put into a food processor or blender and process; otherwise serve as is.

28
Vibrant Vegetables

COOKED VEGETABLES HAVE a marvellous flavour of their own – there's nothing like the crunchy pleasure of a baked potato stuffed with a well-dressed biogenic salad, the light, crisp taste of stir-fried mange-tout spiked with almond slivers, or the spicy tang of a good curry. Each vegetable has its own character and, like a special child, needs to be handled in an individual way to get the most from it.

In this section you will find all sorts of vegetable dishes prepared in many different ways. Some are best used as small side-dishes; others – particularly some of the mixtures – make wonderful meals in themselves and are great for entertaining.

Stir-Fried Vegetables
These attractive and quick vegetable dishes are based on the Chinese principle of frying vegetables very quickly in a minute quantity of light oil. If you're in a hurry, all of your vegetables may be prepared in advance, chopped and left in the refrigerator for when you are ready to cook them.

Each stir-fry recipe is based upon the same principles and there are many different combinations you can try. We stir-fry any vegetables that we can find sitting in the refrigerator. With larger vegetables such as cauliflower florets, the trick is to cut them fine enough so that they can cook within a three-minute period. Here are a few suggestions, but don't be afraid to create your own combinations.

Mange-Tout and Almond Stir-Fry (protein)

A delightful protein dish, thanks to the combination of delicate green mange-tout and crunchy almonds.

8 oz mange-tout
2 tbsp soya oil
2 oz almonds (preferably blanched)
4 oz button mushrooms
1 tsp vegetable bouillon powder

Top and tail the mange-tout. Heat oil in a wok or large frying pan and when hot add the almonds and stir-fry for three to five minutes. Then add the remaining ingredients and continue to stir-fry for another two to three minutes. Serve immediately.

Biogenic Stir-Fry (neutral)

This neutral recipe is based on the biogenic sprouts – whatever sprouts you have will do nicely. Chinese mung-bean sprouts are traditionally used.

2 tsp soya oil
8 oz mung sprouts or *other sprouted seeds or grains*
1 large red pepper, deseeded
1 tsp vegetable bouillon powder or *soy sauce*
black pepper, freshly ground

Heat the oil in a wok or large frying pan. When hot, stir-fry the sprouts and pepper for one to two minutes. Add a little vegetable bouillon powder or soy sauce, season with black pepper, and serve immediately.

Green Stir-Fry (protein)

A lovely protein dish which goes well with a watercress salad.

1 tbsp soya oil
2 oz cashew nuts or *cashew-nut pieces*
2 cloves garlic, chopped finely
8 oz Chinese leaves, shredded
8 oz broccoli florets
8 oz green beans, sliced diagonally

1 tsp vegetable bouillon powder
1 tbsp spring or *filtered water*
juice of 1 lemon

Heat the oil in a wok or large frying pan. When hot, stir-fry the cashews and garlic for two to three minutes. Then add the vegetables and stir-fry for a further three or four minutes. Mix the vegetable bouillon powder with the water and lemon juice and pour over the vegetables and nuts and stir in well. Serve immediately.

Sesame-Courgette Stir-Fry (protein)

A light protein recipe which my 29-year-old son Jesse adores.

2 tsp sesame seed oil or *soya oil*
4 oz sesame seeds
8 oz courgettes
8 sticks of celery
8 oz carrots
1 tsp vegetable bouillon powder or *tamari*

Cut up the vegetables into matchsticks. Heat the oil in a wok or large frying pan. When hot add the sesame seeds and cook at a high heat for one to two minutes until they begin to brown. Then add the vegetables and cook for another two to three minutes. Season with bouillon powder or tamari and serve immediately.

Russian Red Stir-Fry (neutral)

A very light refreshing cabbage dish which is quick and easy to prepare.

3/4 lb red cabbage or *Savoy cabbage*
1/2 lb white turnip
1 tbsp olive oil
4 spring onions, chopped finely
1 tbsp soy sauce
1 tbsp tomato purée
1 tsp cumin seeds
1 tsp paprika
1 tsp vegetable bouillon powder
freshly ground black pepper

Wash the cabbage and shred finely. Grate the turnip finely. Heat the oil in a large saucepan or wok and fry the cabbage–turnip mixture together with the spring onions over a high heat for three minutes. Add the remaining ingredients (including a little spring or filtered water if necessary) and cook for a further five minutes. Season with black pepper and serve immediately.

Other Favourite Vegetable Recipes

Artichokes (neutral)

Artichokes are one of my favourite vegetables. I like them served in almost any form. A simple vinaigrette sauce is perhaps best of all.

4 large artichokes
juice of ¹/₂ a lemon
sea-salt to taste
vinaigrette sauce or *dip* or *seed milk*

Place the artichokes in a large pot of boiling water – at least 3in depth of water. Add the lemon juice and a pinch or two of sea-salt to season, and bring to the boil. Simmer for 45 minutes until the meat at the bottom of each artichoke leaf is softened. Remove and serve either hot or cold with a simple vinaigrette sauce or one of the richer dips or seed milks.

Corn on the Cob (starch)

4 corn-cobs
sea-salt to season
Tahini Mayonnaise dressing (see page 207) or *a little butter and salt*

Remove the corn husks and silk. Place the cobs in boiling, salted water and cook for 10–12 minutes. Strain and serve with Tahini Mayonnaise dressing or a little butter and salt.

Minty Peas (starch)

1 lb fresh shelled garden peas
¹/₂ tsp vegetable bouillon powder
1 tbsp spring or filtered water
2 tbsp fresh mint (apple mint is particularly good)

Put the peas into a pot with the water and vegetable bouillon powder and gently steam over a low heat for 15–20 minutes. Sprinkle with the mint for the last five minutes of cooking and serve immediately.

Pumpkin in Tahini (starch)

The small amount of tahini used here does not interfere with this starch vegetable and sets it off nicely.

1 large onion, chopped finely
1 tbsp olive oil
1 lb fresh pumpkin (skin removed), cut into 1in cubes
1 tbsp tahini
¹/₂ tsp grated nutmeg

Sauté the onion in the oil until brown, then add the pumpkin and continue to sauté for 5–10 minutes, stirring carefully. Add a splash of water if necessary and leave on a very low heat for another 10–15 minutes until soft. Add the tahini and mix well. Serve immediately sprinkled with the grated nutmeg.

Easy Vegetable Curry (starch)

This is a simple and yet delicious dish which takes no more than 20–30 minutes to prepare. It is a good dish to be eaten on its own or with a light salad for supper. In smaller quantities it can be served as a side-dish to go with a biogenic salad.

1 large onion, chopped finely
1 tbsp soya oil or *olive oil* or *sunflower oil*
2 tsp mild curry powder
1–1¹/₂ tsp vegetable bouillon powder
3 large carrots, sliced three or four times lengthways, then cut across to make 1¹/₂in sticks
1 medium-sized turnip, cut up finely into matchsticks
2 potatoes
1¹/₂ C spring or *filtered water*
grated coconut (optional)

Sauté the onion gently in the oil until it becomes translucent, then add the curry powder and vegetable bouillon powder and continue to stir for a few minutes. Add the rest of the vegetables and pour in the water. Bring to the boil and simmer slowly for 20–30 minutes, then serve. It is particularly nice served with some grated dried coconut.

This vegetable curry can be adapted to whatever vegetables you have on hand. During the summer it's delightful to be able to add some French beans or some peas (I often like to add some chopped celery) – or, really, whatever other vegetables you have in the refrigerator.

Spicy Shish Kebab (neutral)

A delicious marinated, skewered vegetable dish which you can grill or barbecue. It is beautiful served on a bed of brown rice which has been cooked with vegetable bouillon powder and herbs. You will need two skewers for each person and it's a good idea to marinate the vegetables for two to four hours.

1 large aubergine, cut into 1¼in chunks
10 fresh tomatoes, halved
24 large mushrooms
1 red pepper
1 green pepper
2 large onions (preferably red), cut into 1in chunks
1 large swede or 2 small turnips, cut into 1¼in chunks

For the Marinade
1¼ C olive oil
juice from 3 lemons
2 tbsp red wine
3 cloves of garlic, crushed
1 tsp coriander, crushed
2 tbsp fresh parsley, finely chopped
½ tsp nutmeg, finely ground
1 tbsp fresh basil (optional)
1 tsp dried oregano

Wash, cut and prepare the vegetables. Place all the marinade ingredients together in a large bowl and mix thoroughly. Grill the aubergine until just soft and add with the rest of the vegetables to the marinade. Let it all sit for two to four hours. Skewer the vegetables, alternating from one to another, and baste them with the marinade as they are grilled or barbecued. May be served with a spicy sauce such as a tahini sauce, mayonnaise or chili sauce.

Aubergine Pâté (protein)

I learned this recipe from a Middle Eastern friend who served it to me once. I had absolutely no idea what I was eating but found it completely irresistible. I have never forgotten the experience. You can vary the taste of aubergine pâté considerably by adding different spices or different extra ingredients but the principles of making it are simple and always the same.

2 medium aubergines
4 cloves of garlic, finely chopped
4 tbsp fresh parsley, finely chopped
1 small onion, chopped finely
½ C tahini
1 tsp vegetable bouillon powder or *other seasoning*
½ tsp ground cumin
pinch of cayenne
1 tbsp olive oil or *Tahini Mayonnaise (see page 207)*

Remove the stems from the aubergines and prick them with a fork as you would a potato. Put them in the oven and bake slowly until they become soft inside. Remove them, then scoop out the insides and put into a food processor to purée. Combine all the other ingredients (except the oil) in the food processor with the purée, remove and chill in a refrigerator. Pour the olive oil on top just before serving. You can use Tahini Mayonnaise instead of the olive oil as a delicious variation.

Vegi-Stroganoff (protein)

A splendid protein-based vegetable dish that can be a real success for entertaining.

2–2½lb chopped fresh vegetables (carrots, celery, courgettes, aubergine, cabbage, Chinese leaves, small tomatoes, cauliflower, broccoli, peas, etc.)

For the Sauce
1½ C raw cashews or *cashew pieces*
1½ C filtered or *spring water (more if needed)*
8 oz chopped mushrooms

1 large onion, chopped finely
1 tbsp soya oil or *olive oil*
juice of 2 lemons
3 tsp vegetable bouillon powder
black pepper
¼ tsp dill
½-1 tsp paprika
3 tbsp dry red wine

To make the sauce you mince the cashew nuts finely in a food processor then add the water and mix further into a creamy consistency. Sauté the mushrooms and onion in the oil until the onion is translucent. Then mix in all remaining sauce ingredients except the red wine. Cook very slowly, either in a double boiler or on a very slow burner. Then steam all the chopped vegetables in a little water. As soon as the vegetables are steamed, which usually takes 20–30 minutes, pour the sauce and wine over them, sprinkle with a dash of paprika and serve immediately.

Ginger Beans (starch)

1 tsp soya or other oil
1 lb French beans
2 cloves garlic, chopped finely
1 tbsp fresh ginger, chopped finely
juice of 1 lemon
1 tbsp tamari or *soy sauce*

Put oil into a wok or large frying pan and heat. When hot, add vegetables, garlic and ginger and stir constantly. Cook for three to four minutes, season with tamari or soy sauce, and serve immediately.

Ratatouille (neutral)

This is a low-fat recipe for ratatouille which makes a delicious main meal. It can be eaten with either a protein or a starch salad. It's very filling.

2 large aubergines
1 large onion

4 cloves of garlic
1 tbsp olive oil
1 tbsp fresh basil or 1 tsp dried basil
1 lb fresh skinned tomatoes or a 15 oz tin of tomatoes
1 large green pepper, deseeded and chopped
6 oz fresh mushrooms
½ lb courgettes, sliced
1 tbsp vegetable bouillon powder
freshly ground black pepper
3 tbsp chopped fresh parsley

Cut the aubergine into ½in cubes; chop the onion and the garlic finely. Heat the oil, then brown the aubergine, onion and garlic in the oil for 5–10 minutes. Add the basil and cook for one more minute, then add tomatoes, green pepper, mushrooms, courgettes and bouillon powder, and simmer for 25 minutes. Season with pepper and sprinkle with parsley. May be served either hot or chilled.

Braised Vegetables (starch)

This simple and inexpensive dish is a favourite with my son Aaron. It combines well with a biogenic salad using a neutral or a starch dressing.

1 head of celery
6 medium potatoes
5 large carrots
2 C spring or filtered water
1 bay leaf
1 tsp vegetable bouillon powder
1 tbsp tahini
freshly ground black pepper

Scrub the vegetables and cut into strips about 3in long. Place in a large pot with water, bay leaf and vegetable bouillon powder; put into an oven pre-heated to 400°F (200°C) Gas mark 6 and bake for 20 minutes. Add tahini and stir well, then replace in oven for a further five minutes. Season with black pepper and serve at once.

Baked Vegetables

I am extremely fond of baked vegetables because the process of baking seems to help the vegetables maintain their natural flavour. Besides, there is something quite charming to me about serving a whole baked onion at a meal: it's amusing as well as delicious.

Baking vegetables is one of the best methods of preserving their vitamins and minerals. You can bake vegetables either on their own or hidden within wholegrain pastry, or you can mix them together in a kind of hot-pot.

Jacket Potatoes (starch)

Baked potatoes make the most wonderful 'pockets' for biogenic salads, bioactive salads, stir-fried vegetables, steamed vegetables and so forth. What you need to avoid are the traditional cheese, sour-cream, yogurt, etc., baked potato fillings because the combination of the starchy potato and the protein of cheese or other dairy products is not a good one. However, there are many neutral vegetables and salads and dips that you can put into baked potatoes, from mashed avocados mixed together with some garlic and a little vegetable bouillon powder to a simple biogenic salad of sprouts with a herbal dressing. One of my most favourite dishes of all is of baked potatoes which have been stuffed with such delicacies.

Pre-heat the oven to 400°F (200°C) Gas mark 6. Scrub the potatoes carefully with a natural bristled brush but do not peel. Pierce the skins two or three times with a fork and bake for 1–1½ hours or until soft. Slit the potatoes open and fill with your desired filling – perhaps a little neutral salad dressing or a little mashed avocado and lemon. Baked potatoes are particularly delicious when sprinkled with fresh parsley which has been chopped finely.

Baked Leeks and Pecans (protein)

1 lb leeks
1 tbsp soya oil or *other cooking oil*
4 oz pecans
2 tbsp miso
splash of spring or *filtered water*

Slice the leeks lengthways in very fine strips and then cut into 3in lengths. Mix well with the oil and bake in a hot oven for 10–15 minutes. Chop the pecans finely in a food processor and combine with the miso and a little water to prepare a sauce for the leeks. Cover the leeks with the sauce and serve immediately.

Baked Carrots (protein)

6 large healthy carrots
1 tbsp olive oil or soya oil
¼ C sesame seeds

Scrub the carrots well and slice them lengthways four or five times, then crossways into pieces about 3in long. Mix well with the oil, then place on a baking sheet and bake in a hot oven for 20 minutes. During the last 10 minutes of baking spread the sesame seeds over the top. Serve immediately.

Baked Parsnips (neutral)

1 lb fresh parsnips
1–2 tbsp sesame oil or olive oil
½ tsp vegetable bouillon powder
2 tbsp Dijon mustard

Slice the parsnips lengthways two or three times, then crossways into lengths about 3in long. Mix together the oil, the vegetable bouillon powder and the mustard and pour over to cover the parsnips. Bake in a moderate oven until golden brown – about 30–35 minutes.

Baked Turnips (neutral)

1 lb fresh turnips
1–2 tbsp oil
1 tsp fresh ginger
½ tsp vegetable bouillon powder
3 tbsp spring or filtered water

Cut the turnips into matchstick-sized strips and put into a casserole with the oil, the finely sliced ginger, the vegetable bouillon powder and the water. Cover with a lid and bake in a moderate oven until tender.

Baked Onions (neutral)

4 large Spanish onions
seed cheese (as dressing)
chopped parsley (as garnish)

Top and tail the onions but leave the outer skin on. Bake in a medium oven for 20–30 minutes until they are yielding to the touch. Take from the oven, remove the outer skins and serve immediately with a seed cheese dressing and a sprinkling of chopped parsley to garnish.

29
Glorious Grains

SIX THOUSAND YEARS ago Zarathustra (Zoroaster), the Persian sage, waxed ecstatic about grains: 'When the light of the moon waxeth warmer,' he said, 'golden-hued grains grow up from the earth during the spring.' I think these words beautifully capture the richness and delight of the grain foods. Grains should always be eaten as close as possible to their natural state. The best way of all to eat them is sprouted. The next best is by cooking them slowly and eating them in side-dishes to go with biogenic or bioactive salads.

The grains are rich in B-complex vitamins. And, providing they are unrefined, they are also rich in fibre. They are excellent foods for providing simple, long-sustained energy – as such, grain dishes play an important part in the diet of athletes. The leaner you become the more you will wish to increase the amount of grains you are eating.

Here are a few simple grain recipes to get you started.

Yummy Brown Rice (starch)

Rice cooked in this manner is so delicious that it seems to be a worthwhile dish in itself. It needs no special sauces or condiments to make it work.

1 C brown rice
2–3 C spring or filtered water
1 tbsp olive oil
2 tsp vegetable bouillon powder
3 tbsp fresh parsley, chopped

1 tsp pot marjoram
2 cloves garlic, finely chopped (optional)

Wash the rice three times under running water and put into a saucepan. Boil the water in a kettle and pour over the rice. Add seasonings except for 1 tbsp of the parsley. Bring to the boil and cook gently for 45 minutes or until all the liquid has been absorbed. Garnish with parsley and serve. (You can double this recipe and prepare enough rice to make a large rice salad the next day.)

Kasha (starch)

A favourite of the Russians, kasha is also a favourite of mine. It is quick to cook and has a pleasant nutty flavour.

2 C buckwheat groats
spring or filtered water to cover
2 tsp vegetable bouillon powder
2 tbsp chopped fresh parsley or other herbs

Place buckwheat in a heavy-bottomed pan and roast it dry over a medium heat while stirring with a wooden spoon. As it begins to darken pour hot water over the buckwheat and add the vegetable bouillon powder and 1 tbsp of the herbs. Cover and simmer very slowly for 15–20 minutes until all the liquid has been absorbed. Serve with the remaining herbs sprinkled on the top.

Polenta (starch)

Polenta is a peasant dish made from cornmeal. I particularly like it served with a biogenic salad dressed with a spicy sauce which I put on the polenta as well.

3 C filtered or spring water
1 C cornmeal
2 tsp vegetable bouillon powder or tamari

Heat the water in a kettle. Pour boiling water over the cornmeal and blend into a paste with the vegetable bouillon powder or tamari. Stir until smooth and cook very gently until all the liquid has been absorbed. Cool and drop by the spoonful onto a slightly oiled baking sheet and grill until brown turning once.

Millet (starch)

Once used by the Romans to make porridge, millet is still an important staple in many parts of Africa. It is a bland and highly nutritious grain which contains all of the essential amino acids plus an excellent complement of the B-complex vitamins and minerals.

5 C spring or *filtered water*
1 C millet
2 tsp vegetable bouillon powder
1 medium onion, chopped finely
1 tsp paprika
2 tbsp chopped parsley, fresh

Boil the water and pour it over the millet in a deep saucepan; then add the vegetable bouillon powder, onion, paprika and half of the parsley. Cook over a slow heat for 30–45 minutes until all of the liquid has been absorbed. Sprinkle with the remainder of the parsley and serve. (Cooked millet can be formed into small balls together with grated carrots, finely chopped onions, a little parsley and a little lemon juice and served cold as part of a salad.)

Barley Pilaff (starch)

A delicious baked dish which goes nicely with a biogenic salad. It is made from pot barley, not from pearl barley (too many of the B-complex vitamins and minerals have been removed from pearl barley). Barley is also excellent used in soups.

2 onions, chopped finely
1 tbsp soya or *olive oil*
1 C pot barley
1½ C spring or *filtered water*
1 tbsp vegetable bouillon powder
1 tbsp dill
2 cloves of garlic, finely chopped (optional)

Sauté the onions in the oil until translucent, then add the barley to the same oil, continuing to stir until the grains have become well coated. Remove from the heat and add the remaining ingredients (including the water, boiled in a kettle). Place in a well-oiled oven dish and bake in a moderate oven for half an hour. Check to see if you need to add a little more water. Serve immediately.

Perfect Oatmeal Porridge (starch)

A superb starch meal and an absolute delight to eat in the evening because the high carbohydrate content of porridge has a tendency to increase the brain's uptake of the amino acid tryptophan and therefore to relax you.

1 C porridge oats
3 C spring or filtered water
pinch of sea-salt
1 ripe banana
1 tsp cinnamon

Preferably soak the oats for several hours before cooking (you can put them in the pot with the water at lunchtime if the porridge is to be prepared for your evening meal). Heat the porridge and water in a double boiler or place the pan containing the oats and water itself in a large frying pan which contains 2in of water. Cook slowly for 15–20 minutes until the mixture has become very smooth. If you prefer a thicker mixture you can reduce the amount of water. Remove from the stove and pour into a dish with sliced bananas and sprinkled with cinnamon. Serve immediately.

30
Out and About

SO THERE YOU have it – the principles, the rationale, the guidelines, the recipes and all the rest. Now it is only a question of putting it all into practice and sitting back to enjoy the transformations that are going to take place in your body. But what about special circumstances? For instance, how do you make biogenics work for you when you have to eat in restaurants, or when you are travelling, or if you want to take your lunch to work or to school with you? It is all a lot easier to cope with than you might imagine.

In a Restaurant
The businessman's lunch or the evening out needn't be a problem. These days more and more restaurants serve decent salads. And, while it is true that most of them are not exactly biogenic delights, they are still a far cry from the traditional limp piece of lettuce with a slice of cucumber, half a tomato and a pale hard-boiled egg.

If you want to eat fish or game then order a dish which is *simply* prepared – not smothered in breadcrumbs (bad starch–protein combination) – such as trout or prawns. If it comes with rice or potatoes ask the waiter if you could please have some vegetables instead and then a mixed or green salad. You can also always order fruit juice or fruit as a starter provided you leave 20 minutes or more before you start on your next course.

If, like me, you prefer most of the time to stick to vegetable foods, you might order a light green salad to start with and follow that with a plate of whatever the vegetables of the day are. The better the restaurant the more helpful they will be. Most of the time you will be able to order without anybody even suspecting that you are practising conscientious food combining.

If, again like me, you prefer to remain as inconspicuous in your dieting as possible, then it is a good idea to order the same number of courses as the other people you are dining with. You could choose an avocado vinaigrette to start with, for instance, followed by a game main course, some vegetables, and a side salad. Nobody will oblige you to eat a sweet these days. I sometimes carry with me some peppermint tea bags as an after-dinner drink while friends are drinking coffee. Then I simply order 'a small pot of tea without the tea please' and pop my bag into it to steep for a couple of minutes when it arrives. By all means enjoy a glass of good wine if you want one.

At Dinner Parties

When I was a child my father always accused me of 'stirring my food around my plate' instead of eating it. He is the only human being I have ever known who actually noticed that I do this. And it is a great technique to practise when you are in a situation where food combinations have been put on your plate which you do not want to eat (this frequently happens to me at dinner parties). The best way to deal with it is to decide whether you are going to make your meal a protein one or a starch one and then eat only the foods in your selected category, simply moving the rest about on your plate so they look well picked over. When your hostess offers you seconds you can reply with, 'Yes I would love some more of that delicious rice,' or 'Do you think I could have another serving of salad; it's wonderful.' At dinner parties make sure you eat plenty of the side-salads, the vegetables and whatever other neutral foods are available. And don't be afraid to say 'no thank you' when people become persistent with their offers. You can always add, 'It looks lovely but I'm afraid I'm rather full.'

On the Go

This is easiest of all. Travelling on planes, in the car or on trains is the ideal time to spend a day on fruit or to applefast. Not only is it convenient, because you have a ready-made opportunity for not following the standard pattern of three meals a day, it will also help your stamina and your ability to withstand the stress of getting from here to there very well indeed. As I've mentioned, I never get on an aeroplane for a long flight without a bag of fruit under my arm. Usually it is the most luscious fruit I can find, since I tend rather to spoil myself on the excuse that 'after all, I'm travelling today and so it's rather a special time'. Most airlines these days offer special meals which fit in well with your needs – for instance, fresh fruit salads with yogurt or cottage cheese, or seafood salads: you need only request them 24 hours before your flight. Once you get used to growing your own sprouts you may even want to carry some of those with you on the go. We often do – especially when we are out hiking (they will grow in plastic bags in a rucksack as well as they do in jars in your kitchen) or when there is a long car journey.

A Packed Lunch

Raw vegetables, fruits or sprouts make excellent foods to put in a lunchbox for school or work. For instance, you can combine any crudités – carrot sticks, celery sticks, broccoli and cauliflower florets, rings or strips of red, yellow and green peppers, mange-tout, diagonal slices of cucumber, courgette, thin slices of Jerusalem artichoke, white radish, kohlrabi, button mushrooms, spring onions, celery hearts, tomatoes, watercress – with a container of seed cheese or a rich protein dressing or dip. This makes a delightful lunch. And, provided you keep your fresh vegetables on hand in the refrigerator all cleaned and ready for use as I do, the whole thing will take you no more than five or ten minutes to prepare.

For most people following a biogenic lifestyle from day to day, being out and about presents little problem. You will probably find after the first few weeks, once you have got the hang of food combining and know pretty well what goes with what, you will not even have to think much about it. After all, if ever things go wrong and you find yourself having eaten a badly combined meal, you can always make the next day an all-raw one or an applefast to get yourself back in balance again.

Happy Ever After

The extraordinary thing about biogenics is that, once you do get into it, once you have shed your unwanted fat, enhanced your energy levels and are feeling in top form, chances are you are going to want to stick with it. When your body has readjusted itself to its normal weight you can begin to experiment a little. Keep to your food combining but now try eating a few more of your foods cooked. Add more grains to your meals. Try the pulses again, for by now your digestive system will probably have become so much more efficient and so much stronger that you will be able to handle them without difficulty. You will see for yourself how easy it is to take everything you have learned together with all the positive changes which have happened to you through new ways of eating and exercising and slowly build for yourself a lasting lifestyle for health and good looks. That, after all, is what biogenics is all about.

References and Further Reading

For Further Information about Biogenics and Useful Recipes

Andrews, Sheila: *The No-Cooking Fruitarian Recipe Book*, Thorsons, Wellingborough, Northants, 1975

Bircher, Dr. Ralph, *et al.*: *Dr Bircher-Benner's Way to Positive Health*, Bircher-Benner Verlag, Zürich, 1967

Bircher, Ruth: *Eating Your Way to Health*, Faber and Faber, London, 1977

Bircher-Benner, Dr. M., and Bircher, Dr. Max: *Fruit Dishes and Raw Vegetables*, C. W. Daniel Co. Ltd, London, 1974

Bircher-Benner Clinic staff: *Bircher-Benner Keep-Slim Nutrition Plan*, Nash Publishing, Los Angeles, 1973

Country Life Restaurant: *Nutrition Seminar Cookbook*, MMI Press, Harrisville, NH, 1984

de Nolfo Jr, Joseph: *No-Cook Recipe Book*, Joseph de Nolfo Jr, Portland, Oregon, 1976

Fathman, G., and Fathman, D.: *Live Foods – Nature's Perfect System of Human Nutrition*, Ehret Literature Pub. Co., Beaumont, Cal., 1973

Gerras, Charles (ed.): *Feasting on Raw Foods*, Rodale Press, Emmanus, Pa., 1980

Grant, Doris, and Joice, Jean: *Food Combining For Health*, Thorsons, Wellingborough, Northants, 1984

Kinz-Bircher, Ruth: *The Bircher-Benner Health Guide*, Unwin Paperbacks, London 1981

Kulvinskas, V.: *Survival Into the 21st Century*, Omangod Press, Wethersfield, Conn., 1975

Livingstone-Wheeler, V., and Wheeler, O. W.: *Food Alive – Man Alive*, Livingstone-Wheeler Medical Clinic, San Diego, Cal., 1977

Nolfi, Dr. Kristine: *My Experiences with Living Food*, Laege F. Skott, Humlegaarden, Denmark, n.d.

Ridgeway, Judy: *Sprouting Beans and Seeds*, Century, London, 1984

Shelton, Herbert M.: *Food Combining Made Easy*, Dr Shelton's Health School, San Antonio, Texas, 1975

Székely, E. B.: *Biogenic Reducing – The Wonder Week*, International Biogenic Society, Costa Rica, 1977

Székely, E. B.: *The Book of Living Foods*, International Biogenic Society, Costa Rica, 1977

Székely, E. B. (ed.): *The Essene Science of Life*, International Biogenic Society, Costa Rica, 1978

Székely, E. B.: *Guide to the Essene Way of Biogenic Living*, International Biogenic Society, Costa Rica, 1977

Székely, E. B.: *The Preventative Diet for Heart and Overweight*, International Biogenic Society, Costa Rica, 1977

Székely, E. B.: *Scientific Vegetarianism*, International Biogenic Society, Costa Rica, 1977

Székely, E. B.: *Search for the Ageless – Vol. 3, The Chemistry of Youth*, International Biogenic Society, Costa Rica, 1977

Thrash, A. M., and Thrash Jr, C. L.: *Nutrition for Vegetarians*, Thrash Publications, Yuchi Pines Inst., Seale, Alabama, 1982

Tobe, John H.: *No Cook Book*, Provoker Press, St Catherines, Ontario, 1979

Walker, Norman W.: *Diet and Salad Suggestions*, Norwalk Press, Wickenbury, Arizona, 1956

Walker, Norman W.: *Pure and Simple Natural Weight Control*, O'Sullivan Woodside and Co., Phoenix, Arizona, 1976

Whyte, K. C.: *The Original Diet*, Troubador Press, San Francisco, 1977

Wigmore, Ann: *The Hippocrates Diet and Health Program*, Avery Publishing Group Inc., Wayne, New Jersey, 1983

Wigmore, Ann: *Hippocrates Live Food Program*, Hippocrates Press, Boston, Mass., 1984

Wigmore, Ann: *Naturama Living Textbook*, Ann Wigmore, Boston, Mass.

Wigmore, Ann: *Recipes for Longer Life*, Rising Sun Publications, Boston, Mass., 1978

Wilson, Frank: *Successful Sprouting*, Thorsons, Wellingborough, Northants, 1978

Chapter One: Lean and Alive

Bircher-Benner, M.: *Food Science For All*, C. W. Daniel, London, 1928

Kenton, L.: *The New Ageless Ageing*, Ebury Press, London, 1995

Kenton, L. and Kenton, S.: *The New Raw Energy*, Vermilion, London, 1995

Precope, John: *Hippocrates in Diet and Hygiene*, Zeno, London, n.d.

Rabagliati, A.: *Human Life and The Body*, C. W. Daniel, London, 1925

Székely, E. B.: *Guide to the Essene Way of Biogenic Living*, International Biogenic Society, Costa Rica, 1977

Waerland, A.: *In The Cauldron of Disease*, David Nutt, London, 1934

Chapter Two: Lean for What?

Bruch, H.: *Eating Disorders*, Basic Books, New York, 1973

Cannon, G., and Einzig, H.: *Dieting Makes You Fat*, Century, London, 1983

Crisp, A. H., and McGuiness, B.: 'Jolly Fat', *British Medical Journal*, I, 1976, 7–9

Glucksman, M., *et al.*: 'The Response of Obese Patients at Weight Reduction', *Psychosomatic Medicine*, 30, 1968, 359–73

Herman, P., and Mack, D.: 'Restrained and Unrestrained Eating', *Journal of Personality*, 43, 1975, 666–72

Kaplan, H., and Kaplan, S.: 'The Psychosomatic Concept of Obesity', *Journal of Nervous and Mental Disease*, 125, 1957, 181–201

Moore, M., *et al.*: 'Obesity, Social Class and Mental Illness', *Journal of the American Medical Association*, 181, 1962, 962–66

Orbach, Susie: *Fat is a Feminist Issue*, Paddington Press, New York, 1978

Orbach, Susie: *Fat is a Feminist Issue 2*, Hamlyn, London, 1982

Rand, Colleen: 'Obesity and Human Sexuality', *Medical Aspects of Human Sexuality*, 13 (Jan 1969), 140–52

Stunkard, A.: 'The Dieting Depression', *American Journal of Medicine*, 23 (1957), 77–86

Stunkard, A.: 'Obesity and the Denial of Hunger', *Psychosomatic Medicine*, 21, 1959, 281–89

Stunkard, A.: *The Pain of Obesity*, Bell Publishing, Palo Alto, 1976

Chapter Three: Calorie-Counting Doesn't Work

'Do The Lucky Ones Burn Off Their Dietary Excesses?', *Lancet*, 2, 1979

Bennett, W., and Gurin, J.: *The Dieter's Dilemma*, Basic Books, New York, 1982

Booth, D.: 'Acquired Behavior Controlling Energy Intake and Output', in Stunkard, A. (ed.), *Obesity, op. cit.*

Boyle, P. C., *et al.*: 'Increased Efficiency of Food Utilization Following Weight Loss', *Physiology and Behaviour*, 21, 1978

Bray, G.: 'Effect of Caloric Restriction on Energy Expenditure in Obese Patients', *Lancet*, 2, 1969

Cannon, G., and Einzig, H.: *Dieting Makes You Fat*, Century, London, 1983

Durnin, J. G. V. A.: 'Energy Balance in Man with Particular Reference to Low Intakes', *Bibliotheca Nutritionis et Dieta*, 27, 1979

Keesey, Richard E.: 'A Set-Point Analysis of the Regulation of Body Weight', in Stunkard, A. (ed.), *Obesity, op. cit.*

Kenton, Leslie: *Lean Revolution*, Ebury Press, London, 1994

Miller, D. S., and Parsonage, S.: 'Resistance to Slimming', *Lancet*, 1, 1975

Mrosovsky, Nicholas, and Powley, T. L.: 'Set Points for Body Weight and Fat', *Behavioral Biology*, 20, 1977

Sjøstrøm, Lars: 'Fat Cells and Body Weight', in Stunkard, A. (ed.), *Obesity, op. cit.*

Chapter Four: Fat Has Its Reasons

Bennett, W., and Gurin, J.: *The Dieter's Dilemma*, Basic Books, New York, 1982

Booth, David A.: 'Acquired Behavior Controlling Energy Intake and Output', in A. Stunkard (ed.), *Obesity, op. cit.*

Bray, George: 'Effect of Caloric Restriction on Energy Expenditure in Obese Patients', *Lancet*, 2, 1969, 397–98

Durnin, J. G. V. A.: 'Energy Balance in Man with Particular Reference to Low Intakes', *Bibliotheca Nutritionis et Dieta*, 27, 1979, 1–10

Enzi, G., *et al.*: *Obesity: Pathogenesis and Treatment*, Academic Press, New York, 1981

Guyton, Arthur C.: *Medical Physiology*, W. B. Saunders, London, 1981

Johnson, D., and Drenick, E. J.: 'Therapeutic Fasting in Morbid Obesity', *Addictive Behavior*, 6, 1981, 155–66

Jung, R. T., and James, W. P. T.: 'Is Obesity Metabolic?', *British Journal of Hospital Medicine*, December 1980

Keesey, Richard E.: 'A Set-Point Analysis of the Regulation of Body Weight', in Stunkard, A. (ed.), *Obesity, op. cit.*

Miller, D. S., and Parsonage, S.: 'Resistance to Slimming', *Lancet*, 1, 1975, 773–75

Mrosovsky, Nicholas, and Powley, Terry L.: 'Set Points for Body Weight and Fat', *Behavioral Biology*, 20, 1977, 205–23

Mueller, William H., and Reid, Russel M.: 'A Multivariate Analysis of Fatness and Relative Fat Patterning', *American Journal of Physical Anthropology*, 50, 1979, 199–208

Nolfi, Kristine: *My Experience with Living Foods*, Humlegaarden, Denmark, n.d.

Rothwell, Nancy, and Stock, Michael: 'A Role for Brown Adipose Tissue in Diet-induced Thermogenesis', *Nature*, 281, 1979, 31–35

Sjøstrøm, Lars: 'Fat Cells and Body Weight', in Stunkard, A. (ed.), *Obesity*, *op. cit.*

Tilden, J. H.: *Toxemia Explained*, Tilden's Health Review and Critique, Denver, Colorado, 1926

Trayhurn, P., *et al.*: 'Thermogenic Defect in Pre-obese ob/ob Mice', *Nature*, 266, 1977, 60–61

Van Italie, T. B., *et al.*: 'Short Term and Long Term Components in the Regulation of Food Intake', *American Journal of Clinical Nutrition*, 30, 1977, 742–57

Walker, Norman W.: *Natural Weight Control*, O'Sullivan Woodside and Co., Phoenix, Arizona, 1981

Williams, R.: *Nutrition Against Disease*, Pitman Publishing Co., New York, 1971

Wirtshafter, David, and Davis, John D.: 'Set Points, Settling Points, and the Control of Body Weight', *Physiology and Behavior*, 19, 1977, 75–78

Chapter Five: Enter the Hero: Biogenics

'A Therapeutic Trial of a Raw Vegetable Diet in Chronic Rheumatoid Conditions', *Proceedings of the Royal Society of Medicine*, Vol. 30, Oct. 1936

Ames, Bruce: 'Dietary Carcinogens and Anticarcinogens', *Science*, Sept. 1983

Bircher, Ralph: 'A Turning Point in Nutritional Science', reprint from *Lee Foundation for Nutritional Research*, 80, Milwaukee, Wisconsin

Bircher, Ruth: *Eating Your Way to Health*, Faber, London, 1966

Bircher-Benner, Max: 'The Meaning of Therapeutic Order', unpublished translation by Hilda Marlin

Bircher-Benner, Max: *The Prevention of Incurable Disease*, James Clarke and Co., Cambridge, 1981

De Vries, Arnold: *The Elixir of Life*, Chandler Book Co., Chicago, 1958

Douglass, J. M., *et al.*: 'Nutrition, Non-thermally Prepared Food and Nature's Message to Man', *Journal of the International Academy of Preventative Medicine*, Vol. 7, July 1982

Evans, R. J., and Butts, H. A.: 'Inactivation of Amino Acids by Autoclaving', *Science*, Vol. 109, 1949

Hein, R. E., and Hutchings, I. J.: *Nutrients in Processed Foods*, ed. American Medical Association on Foods and Nutrition, Publishing Sciences Group, Acton, Mass., 1974

Kenton, L.: *Lean Revolution*, Ebury Press, London, 1994

Pottenger Jr, F. M.: 'The Effect of Heat Processed Foods', *American Journal of Orthodontistry and Oral Surgery*, Vol. 32, No. 8, 1946

Price, Weston: *Nutrition and Physical Degeneration*, Price-Pottenger Nutritional Foundation, La Mesa, Cal., 1970

Priestley, R. J. (ed.): *Effects of Heating on Foodstuffs*, Applied Science Publishers, London, 1979

Székely, E. B.: *The Chemistry of Youth*, International Biogenic Society, Costa Rica, 1977

Székely, E. B.: *Search For The Ageless; Vol. 2: The Great Experiment*, International Biogenic Society, Costa Rica, n.d.

Walker, Norman W.: *Natural Weight Control*, O'Sullivan Woodside and Co., Phoenix, Arizona, 1981

Chapter Six: The Light of Metabolism

Becker, R. O.: 'The Basic Biological Data Transmission and Control Systems Influenced by Electrical Forces', *Annals of the New York Academy of Sciences*, II, Oct. 1974, 238

Becker, R. O.: *Electromagnetism and Life*, State University of New York Press, Albany, n.d.

Bircher-Benner, Max: *Food Energy*, John Bales, Sons and Co., London, 1939

Burr, Harold Saxton, *Blueprint For Immortality*, Neville Spearman, London, 1952

Crile, George: *The Bipolar Theory of Living Processes*, Macmillan, New York, 1926

Kenton, L.: *The New Ageless Ageing*, Ebury Press, London, 1995

Kenton, L., and Kenton, S.: *The New Raw Energy*, Vermilion, London, 1995

Passmore R., and Robson, J. S.: *A Companion To Medical Studies, Vol. I*, J. P. Lippincott and Co., Philadelphia, 1974

Pohl, Herbert A.: 'The AC Field Patterns about Living Cells', in *Cell Biophysics*, Vol. 7, 1985

Pohl, Herbert A.: 'Biological Dielectrophoresis: Applications to the Determination of the Dielectric Properties of Cells, to Cell Sorting, and to Fusion', *IEEE Conference on Elec., Insul. and Dielectric Phen.*, 1982

Pohl, Herbert A.: 'Electrical Aspects of Cellular Reproduction', in E. Clementi *et al.* (eds), *Structure and Motion: Membranes, Nucleic Acids and Proteins*, Adenine Press, 1985

Pohl, Herbert A.: 'The Electrofusion of Cells' *International Journal of Quantum Chemistry: Quantum Biology Symposium*, II, 1984

Pohl, Herbert A.: 'Natural Alternating Fields Associated with Living Cells', in R. K. Mishra (ed.), *The Living State*, World Scientific Press, 1985

Pohl, Herbert A.: 'Natural Oscillating Fields of Cells', in H. Frohlic and F. Kremer (eds), *Coherent Excitations in Biological Systems*, Springer-Verlag, Berlin-Heidelberg, 1983

Popp, F. A.: 'Biophoton Emission – New Evidence for Coherence and DNA Source', in *Cell Biophysics*, Vol. 6, 1984

Popp, F. A.: 'Emission of Visible and Ultraviolet Radiation by Active Biological Systems', in *Proceedings of an International Workshop, November, 1979*, Gordon and Breach Science Publishers, 1979

Popp, F. A.: 'Evidence of Photon Emission from DNA in Living Systems', *Naturwissenschaften*, 68, 1981, 572

Szent-Györgyi, A.: *Introduction to Submolecular Biology*, New York, Academic Press, 1960

Williams, R.: *The Wonderful World Within You*, New York, Bantam Books, 1977

Chapter Seven: Cell Vitality Plus

Bircher, Ralph: 'A Turning Point in Nutritional Science', reprint from *Lee Foundation for Nutritional Research*, 80, Milwaukee, Wisconsin

Bircher-Benner, Max: *The Essential Nature and Organization of Food Energy and the Application of the Second Principle of Thermo-dynamics to Food Value and Its Active Force*, John Bale, Sons and Curnow, London, 1939

Bircher-Benner, Max: *The Prevention of Disease by Correct Feeding*, London, Food Education Co., 1934

Bircher-Benner, Max: *Raw Food In Health and Disease*, Manchester, The Vegetarian Society, 1947

Boyle, P. C., *et al.*: 'Increased Efficiency of Food Utilization Following Weight Loss', *Physiology and Behavior*, 261–274, 1978

Bray, George: 'Effect of Caloric Restriction on Energy Expenditure in Obese Patients', *Lancet*, 2, 1969, 397–98

Drews, J. R.: *Unfired Food and Tropo-therapy*, Chicago, J. D. Drews, 1909

Eimer, Karl: 'Klinik Schwenkenhacher', *Zeitschrift für Ernährung*, July, 1933

Eppinger, Hans: *Die Permeabilitätspathologie als Lehre vom Krankheitsbeginn*, Vienna, 1949

Eppinger, Hans: 'Transmineralisation und vegetarische Kost', in *Ergebnisse der Inneren Medizin und Kinderheilkunde*, Vol. 51, 1936

Eppinger, Hans: 'Über Rohkostbehandlung', *Wiener Klinische Wochenschrift*, No. 26

Gibbin, S.: *Unfired Food in Practice*, C. W. Daniel, London, 1924

Kanai, I.: 'Effects of a Vegetarian Diet, Raw or Cooked, on Oxidation in the Body', *Stschr. F. D. Ges. Exp. Med.*, 89, 131–140

252   The New Biogenic Diet

Karstrom, Henning: *Ratt Kost*, Skandinavska Bokforlaget, Gävle, 1982

Miller, D. S., and Parsonage, S.: 'Resistance to Slimming', *Lancet*, 1, 1975, 773–75

Walker, Norman W.: *Natural Weight Control*, O'Sullivan Woodside and Co., Phoenix, Arizona, 1981

Chapter Eight: Nature's Way to Appetite Control

Abrams, G. D., and Bishop, J. E.: 'Normal Flora and Leukocyte Mobilization', *Archives of Pathology*, Vol. 70, February, 1965, 213–17

Alvarez, Walter C.: 'Enzyme Defects Can Induce Cell Ageing', *Geriatrics*, August, 1970, 72

Bircher, Ralph: *Gesunder durch weniger Eiweiss, Gehmarchiv der Ernährungslehre, Hochsteistungskost für Sport, Berg, Eis, Wüste und Dschungel, Sturmfeste Gesundheit, Hunza das Volk, dass keine Krankheit kannte*, all published in the series 'Edition Wendepunkt', Bircher-Benner Verlag, 1980–81

Dineen, P.: 'Effect of Alteration in Intestinal Flora on Host Resistance in Systemic Bacterial Infection', *Infectious Diseases*, 109, Nov/Dec, 1961

Douglass, J. M., *et al.*: 'Nutrition, Non-thermally Prepared Food and Nature's Message to Man', *Journal of the International Academy of Preventative Medicine*, Vol. VII, No. 2, July, 1982

Hill, M. J., *et al.*: 'Bacteria and Etiology of Cancer in the Large Bowel', *Lancet*, 1, 1970, 95–100

Karstrom, Henning: *Protectio Vitae*, Feb., 1972

Karstrom, Kenning: *Ratt Kost*, Skandinavska Bokforlaget, Gävle, 1982

Virtanen, A. I.: *Angewandte Chemie*, Vol. 70, Nos 17–18, 1958, 544–52

Virtanen, A. I.: 'Die Enzyme in Lebendigen Zellen', *Suomen Kemistilehti*, B. XV, 1942

Virtanen, A. I.: *Report on Primary Plant Substances and Decomposition Reactions in Crushed Plants*, Biochemical Institute, Helsinki, 1964

Virtanen, A. I.: *Suomen Kemistilehti*, 4, 1964, 108–25

Walker, Norman W.: *Natural Weight Control*, O'Sullivan Woodside and Co., Phoenix, Arizona, 1981

Chapter Nine: Digestion and Energy Crisis

Bigwood, E. J.: *Protein and Amino Acid Functions*, Pergamon Press, New York, 1972

Carrington, Hereward: *The History of Natural Hygiene*, Health Research, Monkelhumne Hill, California, 1964

Cinque, Ralph: 'Losing Weight Hygienically', *Health Reporter*, 8, 1983, 5

Goodhart, Robert S., and Shils, Maurice E.: *Modern Nutrition in Health and Disease*, Lea and Febiger, Philadelphia, 1978

Grant, Doris, and Joice, Jean: *Food Combining For Health*, Thorsons, Wellingborough, Northants, 1984

Guyton, Arthur C.: *Textbook of Medical Physiology*, Saunders Publishing Co., Philadelphia, 1981

Norman, Philip N.: 'Food Combinations: An Original Scheme of Eating Based upon the Newer Knowledge of Nutrition and Digestion', *Journal of the Medical Society of New Jersey*, 12, 1924, 375

Passmore, R., and Robson, J. S.: *A Companion to Medical Studies Vol. I*, Blackwell Scientific Publications, Oxford, 1976

Randolph, T., and Moss, R.: *An Alternative Approach to Allergies*, Lippincott & Crowell, New York, 1979

Shelton, Herbert: *Food Combining Made Easy*, Dr Shelton's Health School, San Antonio, Texas, 1951

Shelton, Herbert: *Principles of Natural Hygiene*, Dr Shelton's Health School, San Antonio, Texas, 1968

Stryer, Lubert: *Biochemistry*, W. H. Freeman, San Francisco, 1975

Tilden, J. H.: *Toxemia Explained*, Tilden's Health Review and Critique, Denver, Colorado, 1926

Walker, Norman W.: *Become Younger*, Norwalk Press, Phoenix, Arizona, 1949

Walker, Norman W.: *Natural Weight Control*, O'Sullivan Woodside and Co., Phoenix, Arizona, 1981

Chapter Ten: Food, Sensuous Food

Fletcher, Horace: *Fletcherism: How I Became Young at Sixty*, Athletic Publishers Ltd, London, n.d.

Virtanen, A. I.: *Angewandte Chemie*, Vol. 70, Nos 17–18, 1958, 544–52

Virtanen, A. I.: *Report on Primary Plant Substances and Decomposition Reactions in Crushed Plants*, Biochemical Institute, Helsinki, 1964

Virtanen, A. I.: *Suomen Kemistilehti*, 4, 1964, 108–25

Chapter Eleven: Biogenic Powerhouse

Applegate, W. V., and Connolly, P.: Price-Pottenger Lectures, 1974

Botman, S. G., and Crombie, W. M.: *Journal of Experimental Botany*, 9, 1958, 52

Cancer Control Journal, Sept./Dec. 1970, Los Angeles, California

Curtis, C.: *An Account of the Diseases of India as They Appeared in the English Fleet*, Edinburgh, 1807

Evans, R. J., and Butts, H. A.: 'Inactivation of Amino Acids by Autoclaving', *Science*, Vol. 109, 1949

Hegazi, S. M.: *Zeitschrift für Ernährungswissenschaft*, 13, 1974, 210

Kakade, M. L., and Evans, R. J.: *Journal of Food Science*, 31, 1966, 781

Kirschner, H. E.: *Nature's Healing Grasses*, H. C. White Publications, Riverside, Cal., n.d.

Kohler, G. O.: 'Unidentified Factors Relating to Reproduction in Animals' Feedstuffs', Aug. 8, 1953

Kulvinkas, Viktoras P.: *Nutritional Evaluation of Sprouts and Grasses*, Omangod Press, PO Box 255, Wethersfield, Conn., 1978

Kuppuswamy, S.: 'Proteins in Food', Indian Council of Medical Research, New Delhi, 1958

Maiser, A. M., and Poljakoff-Mayber, A.: *The Germination of Seeds*, Pergamon Press, Oxford, 1966

Price, W.: *Nutrition and Physical Degeneration*, Price-Pottenger Foundation, La Mesa, Cal., 1970

Price-Pottenger Foundation: *The Guide to Living Foods Workbook*, Price-Pottenger Foundation, La Mesa, Cal., 1978

Ridgeway, Judy: *Sprouting Beans and Seeds*, Century, London, 1984

Sellmann, Per, and Sellmann, Gita: *The Complete Sprouting Book*, Turnstone Press, Wellingborough, Northants, 1981

Székely, E. B.: *The Essene Gospel of Peace*, International Biogenic Society, Costa Rica, 1978

Tsai, C. Y., and Dalby, A., *et al.*: 'Lysine and Tryptophan Increases During Germination of Maize Seed', *Cereal Chemistry*, Vol. 52, No. 3, 1975

Chapter Twelve: Headstart – The Applefast

Buchinger, Otto H. F.: *About Fasting*, Thorsons, Wellingborough, Northants, 1983

Carque, Otto: *Vital Facts About Food*, Keats Publishing Inc., New Canaan, Conn., 1975

Ehret, Arnold: *Rational Fasting*, Benedict Lust Publications, New York, 1971

Kadans, Joseph M.: *Encyclopedia of Medicinal Foods*, Thorsons, Wellingborough, Northants, 1973

Kirschman, John D., and Dunne, Lavon J.: *Nutrition Almanac (2nd edition)*, McGraw-Hill, New York, 1984

Koch, Manfred: *The Whole Health Handbook*, Sidgwick and Jackson, London, 1984

Macfadden, Bernard: *Fasting For Health*, Arco Publishing Co. Inc., New York, 1978

Shelton, Herbert M.: *The Science and Art of Fasting*, Natural Hygiene Press, Chicago, 1978

Thrash, A. M., and Thrash, C. L.: *Nutrition For Vegetarians*, Thrash Publications, Yuchi Pines Institute, Seale, Alabama, 1982

Chapter Thirteen: Supplementary Benefits

Borum, P. R., and Fisher, K. D. (eds): *Health Effects of Dietary Carnitine*, Federation of American Societies for Experimental Biology, Bethesda, Md., November 1983

Bremer, J.: *Trends in Biochemical Sciences*, 2, 207–209

Broquist, H. P., and Borum, P. R.: 'Carnitine Biosynthesis: Nutritional Implications', *Advances in Nutritional Research*, 4, Plenum Publishing, New York, 1982

Carroll, J. E., *et al.*: *American Journal of Clinical Nutrition*, 31, 1981, 2693–2698

Frenkel, R. A., and McGarry, J. D. (eds): *Carnitine Biosynthesis, Metabolism and Functions*, Academic Press, New York, 1980

Kenton, L.: *The New Ageless Ageing*, Ebury Press, London, 1995

Kutsky, Roman: *Handbook of Vitamins, Minerals and Hormones, 2nd edition*, Van Nostrand Reinhold, New York, 1981

Leibovitz, Brian: *Carnitine – the Vitamin B_T Phenomenon*, Dell Publishing Co., New York, 1984

McGarry, J. D., and Foster, D. W.: *Proceedings of the National Academy of Sciences*, 72, 1975, 4385–4388

Mitchell, M. E.: *American Journal of Clinical Nutrition*, 31, 1978, 645–659

Mitchell, M. E.: 'Carnitine Metabolism in Human Subjects II. Values of Carnitine in Biological Fluids and Tissues of "Normal" Subjects', *American Journal of Clinical Nutrition*, 31, 1978, 481–491

Stryer, Lubert: *Biochemistry*, W. H. Freeman, San Francisco, 1975

Chapter Fourteen: Eat and Run

'How to Burn up Fat Faster While Maintaining Muscle', *University of California Clip Sheet*, 20 May 1980

American College of Sports Medicine: 'Position Statement, the Recommended Quantity and Quality Exercise for Developing and Maintaining Fitness in Healthy Adults', *Medicine and Science in Sports*, 10 (No. 3), 1978

Bjorntorp, Per: 'Exercise and Obesity', *Psychiatric Clinics of North America*, I, 1978, 691–96

Bortz, Walter M.: 'Effect of Exercise on Aging – Effect of Aging on

256   *The New Biogenic Diet*

Exercise', *Journal of the American Geriatric Society*, XXVIII 2, Feb. 1980, 49ff

Bortz, Walter M.: 'On Disease, Aging and Disuse', *Executive Health*, Dec. 1983

Edwards, H. T., *et al.*: 'The Energy Requirement in Strenuous Muscular Exercise', *New England Journal of Medicine*, 213, 1935, 532–35

Epstein, L., and Wing, R.: 'Aerobic Exercise and Weight', *Addictive Behaviours*, 5, 1980, 371–88

Greene, James A.: 'Clinical Study of the Etiology of Obesity', *Annals of Internal Medicine*, 12, 1939, 1797–1803

Leon, A., *et al.*: 'Effects of Vigorous Walking Program on Body Composition, and Carbohydrate and Lipid Metabolism of Obese Young Men', *American Journal of Clinical Nutrition*, 32, 1979, 1776–87

Margaria, R., *et al.*: 'Energy Cost of Running', *Journal of Applied Physiology*, 18, 1963, 367–70

Moody, D. L., *et al.*: 'The Effect of a Moderate Exercise Program on Body Weight and Skinfold Thickness in Overweight College Women', *Medical Science in Sports*, I (No. 2), 1969

Skrobak-Kaczynski, J., and Anderson, K. L.: 'The Effect of a High Level of Habitual Physical Activity in the Regulation of Fatness During Aging', *International Archives of Occupational and Environmental Health*, 36, 1975, 41–46

Sperryn, Peter: *Sport and Medicine*, Butterworths, London, 1983

Chapter Fifteen: Mysteries of Fat-Burning

Asimov, Isaac: *The Chemicals of Life*, Mentor–New American Library, New York, 1954

Bailey, Covert: *Fit or Fat*, Houghton-Mifflin, Boston, 1978

Coult, D. A.: *Molecules and Cells*, Longman, London and Harlow, 1974

Fisher, Richard B.: *A Dictionary of Body Chemistry*, Granada, London, 1983

Guyton, Arthur: *Medical Physiology*, W. B. Saunders, Philadelphia, 1981

Kenton, L.: *The New Ageless Ageing*, Ebury Press, London, 1995

Passmore, R., and Robson, J. S. (eds): *A Companion to Medical Studies, Vol. I*, Blackwell Scientific Publications, Oxford, 1974

Rose, Stephen: *The Chemistry of Life*, Penguin, London and Harmondsworth, 1979

Sperryn, Peter: *Sport and Medicine*, Butterworths, London, 1983

Stryer, Lubert: *Biochemistry*, W. H. Freeman, San Francisco, 1975

Chapter Sixteen: Your Biogenic Logbook

Bailey, Covert: *Fit or Fat*, Houghton-Mifflin, Boston, 1978
Cannon, Geoffrey and Einzig, Hetty: *Dieting Makes You Fat*, Century, London, 1983
Cooper, Kenneth H.: *The New Aerobics*, Bantam, New York, 1970
Kuntzleman, Charles T.: *Activities*, Wyden, New York, 1978
Moorehouse, L.: *The Physiology of Exercise*, 7th edition, Mosby, St Louis, 1976
Sperryn, Peter: *Sport and Medicine*, Butterworths, London, 1983
Spino, Dyveke: *New Age Training For Fitness and Health*, Grove Press, New York, 1979

Chapter Seventeen: Biogenics in Question

Bircher, Ralph: 'The Question of Protein' (typed paper from author)
Bircher, Ralph: 'A Turning Point in Nutritional Science', reprint from *Lee Foundation for Nutritional Research*, 80, Milwaukee, Wisconsin
Kenton, L.: *The New Ageless Ageing*, Ebury Press, 1995
Kenton, L.: *The New Ultrahealth*, Ebury Press, London, 1995
Kenton, L., and Kenton, S.: *The New Raw Energy*, Vermilion, London, 1995
Pfeiffer, Carl, and Banks, Jane: *Total Nutrition*, Simon and Schuster, New York, 1980
Winick, M.: 'Slow the Problems of Aging and Quash Its Problems – with Diet', *Modern Medicine*, 15, Feb. 1978, 68–74

Resources

Food Processor: Magimix processors are the best available.

Green Drinks: such as Barley; Carrot, Barley & Spirulina; Alfalfa, Barley & Chlorella Juice Concentrates, are available in powdered form from Xynergy, Ash House, Stedham, Midhurst, West Sussex GU29 0PT. Tel. and fax: 0730 813642.

Herb Teas: Some of my favourite blends include Cinnamon Rose, Orange Zinger, and Emperor's Choice by Celestial Seasonings; Warm & Spicy by Symmingtons; and Creamy Carob French Vanilla. Yogi Tea, by Golden Temple Products, is a strong spicy blend perfect as a coffee replacement.

Honey: The Garvin Honey Company have a good selection of set and clear honeys from all over the world. These can be ordered from The Garvin Honey Company Ltd, Garvin House, 158 Twickenham Road, Isleworth, Middlesex, TW7 7LD. Tel: 081 560 7171. The New Zealand Natural Food Company have a fine range of honey, including organic honey, in particular Manuka honey, known for its anti-bacterial effects. The New Zealand Natural Food Company Ltd, Holt Close, Highgate Wood, London, N10 3HW. Tel: 081 444 5660.

Impedance Units: For further information on measuring lean body mass to fat ratio contact: Bodystat Ltd, PO Box 50, Douglas, Isle of Man, IM99 1DG. Tel: 0642 629 571.

Juice Extractor: Moulinex do an inexpensive centrifugal juicer which is good.

Mail Order Organic Foods: Foods such as nuts, seeds, grains, miso, soybean curd, tahini etc. can be ordered from: Freshlands, 196 Old Street, London, EC1V 9FR. Tel. and fax: 081 490 3170. Or Wild Oats, 210 Westbourne Grove, London, W11 2RH. Tel: 071 229 1063.

Marigold Low Salt Swiss Vegetable Bouillon Powder: This instant broth powder based on vegetables and herbs is available from healthfood stores or direct from Marigold Foods, Unit 10, St Pancras Commercial Centre, 63 Pratt Street, London, NW1 0BY. Tel: 071 267 7368.

Nutritional Supplements: Solgar do a good selection of high potency nutritional supplements. For stockists contact Solgar Vitamins Ltd, Solgar House, Chiltern Commerce Centre, Asheridge Road, Chesham, Bucks, HP5 2PY. Tel: 0494 791 691. For lower potency supplements with high bio-availability, Nature's Own do a good range of vitamins and minerals. For stockists contact Nature's Own, 203–205 West Malvern Road, West Malvern, Worcs, WR14 4BB. Tel: 0684 892 555.

Nutritional Analysis: Biolab Medical Unit in central London is a referral centre for Nutritional Medicine. Patients can be referred by their GP or hospital consultant. Doctors can also contact the unit for advice on laboratory investigations and the correction of nutrient deficiencies or imbalances. Biolab Medical Unit, The Stone House, 9 Weymouth Street, London, W1N 3FF.

Personal Trainers: For help with personal exercise you can contact the National Register of Personal Fitness Trainers, Cecil House, 52 St Andrew's Street, Hertford, Herts, SA14 1JA. Tel: 0992 504 336. They will supply you with a list of personal trainers in Britain. However, not all the best people belong to an organization. A personal trainer I highly recommend was my own. He is Welsh champion weightlifter Rhodri Thomas, 90 Cherry Grove, Derwen Fawr, Swansea, SA2 8AX. He is often willing to spend from a weekend to a week or two working out your own personal programme in your own home which he will then monitor and readjust regularly.

Rebounders: mini trampolines available from PT Leisure Ltd, New Rock House, Dymock, Glos. GL18 2BB. Tel: 0531 85888. Fax: 0531 85820.

Sea Plants: such as kelp, dulse, nori, kombu, can be bought from Japanese grocers or macrobiotic health shops, or ordered from Freshlands, 196 Old Street, London EC1V 9FR. Tel. and fax: 081 490 3170. Or Wild Oats, 210 Westbourne Grove, London, W11 2RH. Tel: 071 229 1063.

Soya Milk: There is one sort of soya milk that does not come in aluminium cartons. It is called Bonsoy and is available from Freshlands, 196 Old Street, London, EC1V 9FR. Tel. and fax: 081 490 3170.

Spirulina: the best is from Xynergy, available in good healthfood stores or ordered by post from: Xynergy, Ash House, Stedham, Midhurst, West Sussex, GU29 0PT. Tel and fax: 0730 813642.

If you wish to keep informed of Leslie Kenton's forthcoming books, videos, workshops and other activities, please write to Leslie Kenton, c/o Ebury Press, Random House, 20 Vauxhall Bridge Road, London, SW1V 2SA, enclosing a stamped, self-addressed A4 envelope.

MONTH ONE

Training heart-rate: [ ]

Day	Exercise	Time taken	Pulse-rate afterwards
1			
2			
3			
4			
5			
6			
7			
8			
9			
10			
11			
12			
13			
14			
15			
16			
17			
18			
19			
20			
21			
22			
23			
24			
25			
26			
27			
28			
29			
30			
31			

Waist: in   *Hips*: in   *Left thigh*: in   *Left upper arm*: in
Weight last month: st lb
Weight this month: st lb

MONTH TWO

Day	Exercise	Time taken	Training heart-rate: ☐ Pulse-rate afterwards
1			
2			
3			
4			
5			
6			
7			
8			
9			
10			
11			
12			
13			
14			
15			
16			
17			
18			
19			
20			
21			
22			
23			
24			
25			
26			
27			
28			
29			
30			
31			

Waist: in   *Hips*: in   *Left thigh*: in   *Left upper arm*: in
Weight last month: st lb
Weight this month: st lb

MONTH THREE

Training heart-rate: [   ]

Day	Exercise	Time taken	Pulse-rate afterwards
1			
2			
3			
4			
5			
6			
7			
8			
9			
10			
11			
12			
13			
14			
15			
16			
17			
18			
19			
20			
21			
22			
23			
24			
25			
26			
27			
28			
29			
30			
31			

Waist: in   *Hips*: in   *Left thigh*: in   *Left upper arm*: in
Weight last month: st lb
Weight this month: st lb

MONTH FOUR

Training heart-rate: [ ]

Day	Exercise	Time taken	Pulse-rate afterwards
1			
2			
3			
4			
5			
6			
7			
8			
9			
10			
11			
12			
13			
14			
15			
16			
17			
18			
19			
20			
21			
22			
23			
24			
25			
26			
27			
28			
29			
30			
31			

Waist: in   *Hips*: in   *Left thigh*: in   *Left upper arm*: in
Weight last month: st lb
Weight this month: st lb

MONTH FIVE

Training heart-rate: ⬜

Day	Exercise	Time taken	Pulse-rate afterwards
1			
2			
3			
4			
5			
6			
7			
8			
9			
10			
11			
12			
13			
14			
15			
16			
17			
18			
19			
20			
21			
22			
23			
24			
25			
26			
27			
28			
29			
30			
31			

Waist: in   *Hips*: in   *Left thigh*: in   *Left upper arm*: in
Weight last month: st lb
Weight this month: st lb

MONTH SIX

			Training heart-rate: ☐
Day	Exercise	Time taken	Pulse-rate afterwards

1
2
3
4
5
6
7
8
9
10
11
12
13
14
15
16
17
18
19
20
21
22
23
24
25
26
27
28
29
30
31

Waist: in   *Hips*: in   *Left thigh*: in   *Left upper arm*: in
Weight last month: st lb
Weight this month: st lb

Index

If you have enjoyed this book, you may also be interested in
the following titles by Leslie Kenton:

Published by EBURY PRESS

Lean Revolution	0 09 178415 8	£5.99
Cellulite Revolution	0 09 177532 9	£5.99
10 Day De-stress Plan	0 09 178508 7	£5.99
10 Day Clean-up Plan	0 09 175428 3	£5.99
Raw Energy Recipes	0 09 178470 0	£5.99
Nature's Child	0 09 177836 0	£6.99

Published by VERMILION

The New Ultrahealth	0 09 178515 4	£7.99
The New Ageless Ageing	0 09 178520 0	£7.99
The New Raw Energy	0 09 178510 3	£7.99
The New Joy of Beauty	0 09 178294 5	£8.99
Endless Energy	0 09 177753 4	£9.99

To obtain a copy, simply telephone Murlyn Services on
0279 427203
You may pay by cheque/postal order/credit card and should allow
28 days for delivery.